OXFORD MEDICAL PUBLICATIONS

Practical Ethics for General Practice

Practical Ethics for General Practice

By

Wendy A. Rogers
Department of General Practice, Flinders University,
Adelaide

and

Annette J. Braunack-Mayer
Department of Public Health, University of Adelaide,
Adelaide

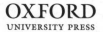

OXFORD
UNIVERSITY PRESS

OXFORD
UNIVERSITY PRESS

Great Clarendon Street, Oxford OX2 6DP

Oxford University Press is a department of the University of Oxford.
It furthers the University's objective of excellence in research, scholarship,
and education by publishing worldwide in

Oxford New York

Auckland Bangkok Buenos Aires Cape Town Chennai
Dar es Salaam Delhi Hong Kong Istanbul Karachi Kolkata
Kuala Lumpur Madrid Melbourne Mexico City Mumbai Nairobi
São Paulo Shanghai Taipei Tokyo Toronto

Oxford is a registered trade mark of Oxford University Press
in the UK and in certain other countries

Published in the United States
by Oxford University Press Inc., New York

A catalogue record for this title is available from the British Library

ISBN 0 19 852504 4 (Pbk)

10 9 8 7 6 5 4 3 2 1

Typeset by Integra Software Services Pvt. Ltd, Pondicherry, India
Printed in Great Britain
on acid-free paper by Biddles Ltd., Guildford and King's Lynn

My recompense is thanks, that's all,
Yet my good will is great, though the gift small.

William Shakespeare
Thaisa, in Pericles

For Peggy and Andy and for Erik, Jakob, Lydia, and Anna.

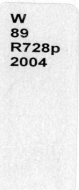

Preface

Twenty years ago, Roger Higgs and I wrote a short book entitled, *In that case: medical ethics in everyday practice* [1]. In it, we expressed the hope that medical ethics would abandon its obsession with the dramas of hospital medicine, and begin to show the relevance of ethics to every facet of medical practice. To illustrate this, we told the story of a fictional patient, "Angie", tracing her odyssey through medical and social agencies to an ending, which may not have been ideal, but which was meant to reflect the continuing moral uncertainty of real life, and, in that, the centrality of trust.

It is refreshing to discover a new book, all these years later, which locates itself firmly in such day-to-day experiences of patients and their general practitioners, and which recognizes the special features of the relationship that general practice makes possible: a relationship with the whole patient, not just a cluster of symptoms; which potentially extends over years; and which recognizes the family and social setting of the patient. Of course, such a richness of relationship is an ideal of general practice, which cannot always be fulfilled. Patterns of practice are changing, as governments seek to influence the way that health care is delivered, and as practitioners rightly seek to protect their personal and family lives. Increasingly, practitioners may rely on the data on their computer screen to understand the full history of a patient, since group practice arrangements often mean that the patient is seen by a series of doctors. Home visits are becoming much less common, and the increasing use of after-hours on-call services often means that the person seeing the patient in an emergency is not their usual daytime practitioner. Despite these

[1] Campbell, A.V. and Higgs, R. (1982). *In that case: medical ethics in everyday practice.* Darton, Longman and Todd, London.

changes, the concept of a generalist or family practitioner, seeing the patient in non-emergency situations in the community, remains the pivotal point for any effective health service. Without it, the ideal of whole-person care will be lost, and the vital importance of preventive medicine and early intervention will be overlooked. We need everyday medical practice and, with it, everyday ethics.

This book offers itself as an easily accessible resource for such ethics. It should sit on the shelf of every doctor's consulting room, alongside the manuals of therapeutics and prescription. In the midst of the pressured life of modern general practice, Wendy Rogers and Annette Braunack-Mayer provide a haven of good sense and practicality. They tease out the common ethical dilemmas of daily practice from a set of fictional vignettes of encounters with patients, which will be instantly recognizable to all practitioners. They are not afraid to provide some answers, as well as raising questions (the favoured activity of philosophers), but there is no "dumbing down" in this book, no dodging of the real complexities and uncertainties of some of the dilemmas patients and practitioners face. Each chapter offers a set of references for further reading into some issues, and the book concludes with a useful guide to the scholarly resources in medical ethics that are currently available.

Arguably, the most important part of the whole book is the closing chapter, 'On being a good doctor'. With its account of virtue ethics, this chapter emphasizes what patients have always known. We need doctors who keep up to date with their knowledge and skills and who remain scientifically active and innovative in the management of their practice. We need doctors who recognize the ethical and legal complexities of the wide range of situations they have to deal with. But beyond this, we need doctors with integrity and compassion. In medicine, as in other professions where one's personal life is exposed and trust is essential, it is the singer, not just the song that matters.

Alastair V. Campbell
Professor of Ethics in Medicine
University of Bristol
Bristol

Acknowledgements

We are indebted to many people for their thoughtful comments, suggestions, ideas, clinical cases, and discussions at various stages in the preparation of this book. In particular, we would like to thank Susan Buck, Jillian Creasy, Patti Gardener, Miriam Santer, Chris Salisbury, Chris Watkins, and members of the Centre for Ethics in Medicine at the University of Bristol, the Departments of General Practice at the Universities of Edinburgh and Adelaide and Flinders University, and the Department of Public Health at the University of Adelaide.

Wendy Rogers wrote drafts of several chapters while on a Sidney Sax fellowship funded by the National Health and Medical Research Council of Australia, hosted by the Department of General Practice at the University of Edinburgh. Annette Braunack-Mayer prepared drafts of chapters while a Visting Research Fellow at the Centre for Ethics in Medicine at the University of Bristol. Both places provided supportive and intellectually challenging environments in which to write. The University of Adelaide provided generous support for Annette's time in the United Kingdom.

We would also like to thank the GPs, patients and students who have participated in our research and teaching endeavours through the years, and whose views and insights have helped to shape our ideas.

Our Australian families followed us to the United Kingdom. Thanks to Matthew Millar and Sarah and David Pearce for their support during our Edinburgh sojourn. Erik, Jakob, Lydia, and Anna Braunack-Mayer accepted the challenge of a Bristol winter and helped create a home in a strange place. For their patience and encouragement during the writing of this book and, particularly, their comments on the cover, we are grateful.

Contents

List of abbreviations

BMA	British Medical Association
EBM	Evidence-based medicine
GMC	General Medical Council
GP	General practitioner
GPC	General practitioners Committee
HF&EA	Human Fertilization and Embryology Act
IVF	In vitro fertilization
MIDIRS	Midwives Information and Resource Service
NHS	National Health Service
NICE	National Institute for Clinical Excellence
QALY	Quality Adjusted Life Year
RCGP	Royal College of General Practitioners

Introduction

General practice is at the heart of health services around the world. GPs are the point of first contact for patients, and the conduit through which other forms of medical care may be accessed. They have multiple obligations—to patients in their care, to government for responsible use of resources, to communities for the standard of health services provided. Ethics is also at the heart of health services, because ethics deals with fundamental questions about what ought to be valued, including health and health services, and why we ought to value particular things. In this book we bring together these two 'hearts' in a textbook on practical ethics for general practitioners.

This book has three main aims. First, we wish to help GPs appreciate the ethically significant nature of general practice, and to draw attention to the ethical complexity of apparently mundane and everyday experience. Many of the issues and cases we discuss will be familiar to GPs and, in some cases, they may appear to raise little of ethical importance at all. We want, first and foremost, to raise awareness of the fact that ethics pervades all areas of general practice.

Secondly, we want to present a thoughtful and thought provoking account of the moral foundations of general practice. In recent years there have been a number of texts published on the philosophy of medicine (Pellegrino and Thomasma 1981; Veatch 1981). While these texts identify and analyse a number of key concepts for ethical practice, their need to cover the breadth of medical practice does not allow them to focus on how these concepts are worked out in specific settings. In this book we explore the ways in which moral concepts such as trust, beneficence, respect for autonomy, and fairness take on particular meanings in the general practice setting.

Our intentions in this book are not only philosophical. We also aim to discuss some specific ethical issues in detail, with a view to offering solutions that are practical, as well as ethically sound. Ethical analysis is occasionally accused of being too abstract and abstruse to be of much value in the real world of messy problems and difficult decisions. Contrary to this view, we want to show how moral concepts and arguments can illuminate murky situations, thus providing a way forward or clarifying a response.

Practical Ethics for General Practice is primarily written for GPs, GP registrars, and students. With this audience in mind, we have tried to ground our description and analysis of ethical concepts in the everyday reality of general practice. Generally, our approach is to introduce a topic with cases, and to define and conceptualize moral concepts in the context of these examples. One of the difficulties with a case-oriented approach to ethics is that the cases can become too 'thin', offering too little detail and losing the charm of realism (Davis 1991). 'Thick' cases, by contrast, provide rich and full descriptions of the detail of cases, but do so at the risk of invading the privacy of individuals who constitute the case. We have attempted to guard against these twin difficulties by drawing our cases from our own experiences and the experiences of our colleagues and friends. Many of the cases had their origins in real life, however all cases have been fictionalized in terms of people, places, and events to protect privacy. Our cases are set in four imaginary general practices, with the same GPs, and sometimes the same patients, reappearing in a number of chapters. We hope this way to paint a more detailed picture of the GP and his or her work, so that, by the end of the book, the reader has some feel for what these GPs value and how they routinely approach moral problems in their work. We introduce our GPs in the following paragraphs.

The GPs and their practices

The Hackney Road Practice, London

The Hackney Road Practice is a large, modern practice in an inner suburb of London. The neat and well-kept exterior of the practice is a contrast to the poverty and deprivation that surrounds it, for the practice serves a particularly poor and underprivileged community with a high proportion of immigrants from African and South East Asian countries.

The Hackney Road Practice has five GPs working in it, but our attention centres on Dr Jeremy Chu and Dr Malcolm Carter, both in their late 30s, who have been in practice here for 10 years. With 25% of his patients HIV positive, Dr Chu has developed an interest in HIV medicine, particularly in the management of AIDS in primary care settings. Over time, he has assembled a team of nurses, health visitors, psychologists, and social workers with expertise in this area. Dr Carter has no special interests. He enjoys general practice, but thinks he would be just as happy in any number of other occupations. Generally, the partners get along well, although there are, as we shall see, occasional differences of opinion as to how the practice should be run.

The Pembroke Crescent Practice, Yorkshire

The Pembroke Crescent Practice is the only practice in Fetways, a small village in Yorkshire. Dr Jack Day has been here for 25 years now, and he and his wife, Joan, are absolutely committed to the village and the practice. Over the years, Dr Day has had a series of assistants. Few stay more than a few years; his last assistant recently moved on and Dr Mira Shah has just joined the practice. This is Dr Shah's first position since completing her general practice training in York. She expects to enjoy the work, but she is apprehensive about the relative isolation of Fetways.

The Westminster Surgery, Bath

The Westminster Surgery is in an attractive, tree lined street in central Bath. The senior partners, Dr John Bowler and Dr Oliver Whittaker, have built the practice up over the years, and it now has an excellent reputation as a training practice. Dr Bowler, at 63, has begun to think about scaling down his work commitments. With this in mind, and to provide a better service for female patients of the practice, the practice employed Dr Imogen Jones a few years ago. Dr Jones has worked part-time since the first of her two children was born three years ago.

The Gordon Road Surgery, Glasgow

The Gordon Road Surgery is a large group practice in outer Glasgow. It has six GPs, including two we will meet in this book. Dr Fiona MacFarlane, a native Glaswegian, is in her early 40s. She has been at Gordon Road for 15 years, and she has a particular interest in women's health. Dr David Grainger has only been with the practice for three years. Now in his early 50s, his career path has been rather unusual, beginning with a science degree, a PhD in physics and research work, and followed by his return to study medicine in his late 30s.

The final GP character in our book is Dr Martin Schroeder. Dr Schroeder originally trained in Berlin, and has worked in Britain for five years now, mainly as a locum. He enjoys locum work, as it provides the flexibility that allows him to travel regularly.

Practical Ethics for General Practice is organized around a number of key ethical concepts. We begin with a discussion of the distinguishing features of general practice, its ethical complexities, and the role of ethics and ethical theory in this milieu. In Chapter 2, we turn to an analysis of the doctor–patient relationship and explore the centrality of trust to that relationship. The latter part of the chapter deals with problems with trust and difficult relationships between doctors and patients.

The promise of confidentiality is one of the ways that GPs make trust explicit. Chapter 3 builds on our discussion of trust with an account of the meaning, importance, and limits to confidentiality.

The obligation to act beneficently—for the good of patients—is central to ethical general practice. However, working out what we mean by the good of the patient, treading the fine line between beneficent and paternalistic actions, and defining the place of evidence in good medical practice, are all issues for the GP who would be beneficent. We explore the concept of beneficence and its extent and limitations in Chapter 4.

The private face of beneficence is in the consulting room, as GP and patient meet together. The public face is more often found in debates and discussion about resource allocation. Chapter 5 explores the issues associated with allocating resources fairly in a general practice setting. We begin with a definition of resource allocation and a description of the ways in which resources are currently allocated in the NHS. This is followed by an account of theories and principles for the fair distribution of resources in general practice.

In Chapter 6 we return to ethical issues that arise mainly in the context of the relationship between GP and patient with a discussion of autonomy and decision-making in general practice. We examine the meaning and importance of autonomy, the nature of informed consent, some limits to autonomy, and the relationship between autonomy and responsibility.

Looking after patients at the beginnings and endings of life provide some of the most difficult and yet most rewarding moments in general practice. Chapters 7 and 8 deal with ethical issues that arise at these points in time. In each chapter we draw on principles and theories that have been laid out in preceding chapters, considering the ways in which respectful decision-making and considering the best interests of those involved can shape choices and practices at these stages of life.

Chapters 2–8 are principally about the ethical issues that arise out of GPs' relationships with patients. Yet, many aspects of GPs' work are not undertaken directly with patients. On a daily basis, GPs interact with patients' families, doctors and other health care professionals, students, industry representatives, government officials, and their own families. In Chapter 9 we explore the ethical issues that arise out of GPs' multiple obligations, using the concept of conflicts of interest.

In the final chapter we revisit the issues we flagged in Chapter 1— 'What is general practice?' and 'What is ethically significant about it?' We discuss the idea of being a good general practitioner, and we draw on insights from virtue theory to integrate motives and character into our account of ethical experience in general practice.

This brief description of the content of *Practical Ethics for General Practice* provides an indication not only of what the book is about, but also of what it is not about. First, we are not driven by an allegiance to any particular school of philosophical thought, and we would regard ourselves as philosophically eclectic. We have not set out to prepare an ethics workbook for general practitioners, although we hope that GP trainers, GPs, and students will all use the book in both formal and informal education. Nor have we been concerned specifically to develop a philosophy of general practice, although there are elements in the book that point in this direction. Finally, *Practical Ethics for General Practice* is not a medico-legal textbook or a code of professional conduct, although there is obviously considerable overlap between the requirements and constraints imposed by the law and professional codes and the ethical practice of medicine. Instead, we have tried to focus attention on the contribution that ethics and ethical reasoning can make to good practice. We hope that this book will provide the impetus for much good discussion, learning, and activity in general practice.

References

Davis, D.S. (1991). Rich cases. The ethics of thick description. *Hastings Center Report* **21**, 12–17.

Pellegrino, E.D. and Thomasma, D.C. (1981). *A philosophical basis of medical practice*. Oxford University Press, New York, NY.

Veatch, R.M. (1981). *A theory of medical ethics*. Basic Books, New York, NY.

Chapter 1

General practice and ethics

Introduction

> The generalist cannot take refuge in the limitations of his specialty. For him the healing relationship must be entered in the fullest sense ... He must help, care for, comfort and ease when the specialist has nothing to offer ... The patient often has made the rounds of the specialties; he is still ill, still needing answers to the key clinical questions. Even if the patient's illness has been 'negotiated' out of medicine by other physicians, someone must remain who can help.
>
> The generalist, on this view, is the physician par excellence since he has the most intimate relationship with the healing and helping functions of medicine. A specialist, especially if his domain is a technique, might get away with only scientifically right decisions; but a generalist, never.
>
> Pellegrino 1983, p. 166

General practice occupies a unique place within medicine. It lies at the heart of the National Health Service, through universal registration with general practitioners, as one of the first points of access for anyone seeking medical care, and as the route to specialist or hospital care. As a discipline, general practice is relatively young; its professional colleges and academic departments formed in the 1950s and 1960s. Since then, there has been increasing attention turned towards the nature of general practice, focusing on clinical methods, philosophy, and research (McWhinney 1997; Starfield 1998). Despite the difficulties of defining general practice, there are a number of points of agreement about the features that distinguish general practice from other branches of medicine. In this chapter, we briefly discuss some of the central features of general practice, and examine their ethical implications. In the second half of the chapter, we offer a brief introduction to ethical terminology and reasoning which will underpin the material in the rest of the book.

The GP–patient relationship

The relationship between GP and patients is a central distinguishing feature of general practice. Pellegrino draws our attention to this relationship in the quote above: in his words the relationship must be 'entered in the fullest sense', from the beginning of the patient's problems through to the exit of the last specialist. The commitment to the patient as a person is prior to any particular health problem that the patient may have. Once a patient is accepted onto a list, the GP is committed to providing care to that person, whether they attend the surgery frequently or infrequently, in good or ill health.

The centrality of the relationship leads directly to many of the other defining features of general practice. The commitment to the patient as a person, irrespective of their state of health, requires a holistic approach to patient care. This may be described in terms of the biopsychosocial model of health, often approached in practice through patient-centred techniques. The main point is that general practice prides itself on seeing its patients first as people, with hopes, fears, lives, jobs, families, and relationships, over and above any health problem that may be presented at the surgery. Specialists may rely on their adeptness at various techniques and fulfil their medical obligations to patients with little interest in or knowledge of their patients' lives, but for general practice, the person comes before the disease. An ophthalmologist, for example can effectively treat an acute penetrating eye injury in a female patient without knowing much about the patient or her life, discharging her once the injury is stable. For her GP, that injury may be one more in a succession of domestic 'accidents', but maybe this is the injury that will lead to disclosure about her violent partner and provide the opportunity for the GP to offer help that will be accepted on this occasion.

This commitment can be a double-edged sword. On one hand, knowing and understanding the circumstances of one's patients can help both diagnostically and therapeutically.

Case 1.1

Ms Jackie Silvers is a 35-year-old mother of three young children. She lives with her husband who is an executive with a computer company and who spends a lot of time away from home. Their youngest child has severe asthma, and the middle child has extremely aggressive behaviour that has responded only poorly to a series of appointments with a psychologist. Ms Silvers presents on this occasion with recurrent headaches. Dr Whittaker knows that her husband is away in the USA on a three week trip, and that the youngest child was admitted last week as an emergency with his asthma. Ms Silvers has recently had a promotion in her work and is now managing a team of staff in the local council offices.

Dr Whittaker takes a history and examines Ms Silvers. His provisional diagnosis is that these are tension headaches, exacerbated by recent stresses in Ms Silvers' life.

In this case, Dr Whittaker's knowledge of Ms Silvers as a person, coupled with a thorough history and examination help him to reach a diagnosis and to spare her the inconvenience and anxiety of further investigations. He is able to help by explaining the likely association between the headaches and her current situation, and suggest practical ways for Ms Silvers to manage her own stress and the children's problems.

Sometimes however, the commitment to a holistic approach and to the patient as a person can be challenging, especially when that person follows a course of action that we do not agree with, or, like the victim of domestic violence, is unable to acknowledge the real problem or accept help. In these cases, the GP cannot walk away from the relationship, but is committed to offering whatever care can be negotiated with the patient at that moment in time. The frustrations of missed opportunities, ongoing damage to health, and limited scope for action can be demoralizing.

This leads us to the next feature of the GP–patient relationship; it continues over time rather than being limited to discrete illnesses. This continuity itself feeds into the relationship, as it allows GPs to know their patients in sickness and in health. The prostrate figure lying vomiting in a dark room with a migraine headache may on another day be a cheerful and confident gardener who has come in for a tetanus injection. Episodic care over time allows both GP and patient to build up their knowledge of each other, and as we discuss in Chapter 2, this is fundamental to the growth of trust in the relationship. Again, the ongoing nature of the relationship can be both rewarding and challenging. Looking after pregnant women, and later their children, or following up a patient after a serious illness are some of the joys of ongoing care. On the other hand, the prospect of years of appointments with patients who have problems that seem insoluble can be daunting.

The comprehensive nature of general practice means that for GPs, surprise is a constant companion. Patients may present with something as routine as an upper respiratory tract infection, or as rare as vacation-acquired tropical disease. The tension headaches may become sinister in nature, or the recurrent complaint of tiredness be due to anaemia rather than depression. Problems may be physical, psychological, or social; they may be amenable or refractory to diagnosis; and there may or may not be something that the GP can do about them. Whatever problems patients bring to their GPs, a response is required; the GP is expected to do something. Even if the patient does not present with a problem, the GP is expected to carry out preventive care.

As well as relationships with individual patients, GPs may also have relationships with families. Of course, not all members of a family necessarily register at the same practice, but often a GP will have more than one family member on their list. Again, this can be helpful in terms of understanding the person who is the patient on this occasion, and the way that the illness is likely to impact upon both the family and the person.

There are two final features about general practice that affect the GP–patient relationship. The first is the location of general practice, in the community in small self-contained surgeries. In comparison with hospitals, general practice surgeries are less intimidating and offer a greater promise of intimacy. Surgeries are often close to people's homes, so that there can be a shared knowledge and understanding of the community. The GP will know if there is adequate (or any) public transport, or if the local factory or school is closing down. Consultations may take place in the patient's home, providing GPs with sometimes invaluable insights into the lives of their patients. This proximity between the medical and the domestic spheres is rare in other branches of medicine.

Finally, general practice is usually the first point of access for patients seeking medical care. Some patients present straight to hospital with emergencies, and some use drop in centres and NHS hotlines, but for most patients it is a visit to the GP that heralds any episode of health care. This means that GPs become familiar with the full range of symptoms that trigger a visit to the doctor, as well as becoming familiar with the variations in threshold that lead some patients to consult only when in extremis while other consult more readily. If a problem is beyond the expertise of the GP, or if further tests or therapies are required, it is the GP who acts as gatekeeper to secondary and tertiary care. And it is to the GP that the patient returns after colleagues in other specialties have made their contributions to the patient's care.

Ethical complexities in general practice

What are the ethical implications of the features of general practice that we have outlined above? Perhaps the most significant feature is that general practice is ethically complex. The GP–patient relationship means that GPs are often closer to their patients and their patients' lives than doctors working in other medical specialities. The closeness of this relationship can lead to insights into ethical values that would not be obvious in other settings. One of the central debates in medical ethics concerns finding the right balance between acting for the good of the patient and respecting patient's rights to self-determination (Christie and Hoffmaster 1986). The ethical terms for these two values are beneficence and autonomy. Historically, acting for the good of the patient has been the dominant value in medicine. Over the past fifty years this has changed, with recognition of the rights of patients to have a much greater say in their treatment.

In many branches of medicine, there can be a quite stark demarcation between these values, with the medical view of what is good for the patient competing with the patient's own view of what is good for them. In general practice, there is far more opportunity to know the patient as a person above and beyond their illness, so that the medical view about the right thing to do becomes influenced by the GP's knowledge of the patient and what is important to them. We pick up this issue in detail in Chapter 4.

GPs' views about the autonomy of their patients are also influenced by their personal knowledge about their patients' lives and circumstances. Rather than having to make an assessment of the patient's capacity for self-determination at one point in time (for example in hospital before an operation, or in a rushed out-patient clinic appointment), GPs are able to form a detailed picture of their patients' lives and develop a greater understanding of the ways that their circumstances influence the choices that they are able to make. The traditional medical ethics view of respecting autonomy is that if patients are fully informed, have a good understanding of the information necessary to make a decision, and are not coerced, then any decision they make is autonomous and should be respected by the doctor. (Patient autonomy is discussed in detail in Chapter 6.) But for general practice, this seems unduly narrow. GPs are able to assess the wider context and to look for factors in their patients' lives that might shape the decisions that seem possible (Doyal 1999). A doctor in an out-patient clinic might accept an elderly woman's decision to refuse an operation for a hip replacement as an autonomous decision, as long as the patient is informed and understands the implications of her decision. For her GP, who knows that the patient is worried about who might look after her frail husband while she is in hospital and recovering from the operation, the decision might appear in a different light. Rather than accepting her decision to forego surgery, the GP would be able to use his relationship with the woman to explore the barriers to surgery, and to ensure that her decision is based upon her own preferences rather than driven by circumstances that she finds overwhelming.

Confidentiality is a key issue in medical ethics. The ethical requirements are straightforward: information about patients should not be divulged to any one else except in quite strictly regulated circumstances. (These are discussed in Chapter 3.) For doctors working in hospitals removed from the communities where their patients live, it is not difficult to maintain confidentiality. For GPs, who are often looking after multiple members of families, keeping information private can be challenging. What if one person's medical information has implications for the health of other members of the family? A woman might see her GP complaining of tiredness and difficulty coping with her elderly father whose behaviour is becoming erratic. She might think that the problems in coping with her father are due to a recurrence of her depression, which she has had in the past. The GP, however, may be aware that the father's behaviour is due to cerebral secondaries from a disseminated cancer, information that the father does not want his daughter to know. The ethical obligation to maintain confidentiality can be difficult if the GP is witness to the distress that secrecy can sometimes cause in families.

The nature of the GP–patient relationship, and the GP's role as gatekeeper to the rest of the health service, mean that patients often rely heavily on GPs to be their advocates. This can create an open-ended commitment—where should GPs draw the line in advocating for their patients? For doctors in other specialities, it is possible to look after patients within the boundaries of their speciality, and to withdraw once those limits are reached. In general practice, medical problems merge into social problems. There is no clear boundary line; many problems are neither clearly within nor outside the medical domain. In addition, GPs are aware of the struggles that patients may have dealing with the NHS or other welfare agencies, and know that unless they help, the patient is likely to struggle unsuccessfully.

The advocacy role, together with open access to general practice, mean that GPs often face unrealistic moral demands (Doyal 1999). How can they meet the needs of their patients when there is barely enough time to see everyone who wants an appointment, when many of their patient's problems are the result of social rather than physiological processes, and when their patients are competing with other patients for scarce resources? And how can GPs be fair in their gatekeeping role while trying to be advocates for their patients?

Finally, the way that general practice is organized means that GPs are often quite isolated. The opportunities for ethical discussion are limited, either because there is no one with whom to discuss ethical issues, or there is no time to do so, given the multitude of pressures on GPs' time. This isolation can magnify ethical complexities, making dilemmas appear insoluble.

Approaches to ethical reasoning

So far we have used the terms 'ethics' and 'ethical' with no discussion or explanation. What do we mean when we say that general practice is ethically complex? One way to answer this question is to say that, for the reasons that we have outlined above, it is difficult to answer the question: 'What is the right thing to do in this situation?' Broadly speaking, ethics deals with the decisions and choices that we make in our lives. The first questions in ethics often may be: 'What should I do in this situation?', or 'What would a good GP do here?' Often there is little doubt about how to respond to these questions and, for the most part, we don't even think about our responses. A patient hobbles in with a sprained ankle—we strap it and prescribe painkillers and rest. Another patient bursts into tears in the consulting room—we reach for the tissues and try to console her. Such responses may seem straightforward. We do not usually stop to consider why we are acting in this way, still less analyse our responses in ethical language. In much of general practice care, ethics drops out of view and we do not think something like: 'I was acting beneficently towards the patient with a sprained ankle.'

Sometimes however, there can be doubt about how to respond. Should I hospitalize this patient with end-stage renal failure? Should I push this wavering mother, so that she will decide to have her children vaccinated today? What are my responsibilities when a patient's family thinks I am doing the wrong thing for their relative? What do I do when a patient asks me to do something I don't want to do? In these situations our confusion may arise because we can envisage more than one appropriate action, or because no action seems quite right.

In both the clear and the confusing cases, ethical deliberation involves further questions that try to uncover our reasons and the values that lie behind those reasons. Why should I help someone with a sprained ankle? Because I have the skills to help, and my treatment will stop the patient from suffering pain, and help to restore them to good health. We can take the questions further: why is it good to reduce suffering, and why do we think that health is so important? The role of ethics is to uncover the reasons that lie behind our assumptions and habits, and to analyse these reasons through a moral lens. This can help us to fashion systematic ways to respond to the choices we face. Ethical reflection provides a way to clarify our values, and to impose some consistency on the confusion of our moral lives.

Ultimately the ethical question is always a 'why' question, for two reasons. First, ethical reasoning is most often invoked when we cannot see a straightforward answer to the question: 'What is the right thing to do?' If we do not know what the best choice is in a situation, it seems fairly obvious that we then examine why certain choices might be better or worse than others, and to look at the deeper values that lead us to those judgements. However, even when we do know what ought to be done, ethics has an important role in making explicit the taken-for-granted assumptions that underpin our actions. Reflecting on mundane and routine decisions helps us to identify the values guiding our decisions, and allows us the opportunity to reconsider these.

Ethics usually comes up in medical discussions when doctors are faced with an ethically difficult decision, and want to know what to do. Doctors often want specific answers to specific problems. But, ethics and ethical reasoning will not always provide an answer for each unique and individual situation. There is no medical ethics rule book that will identify the right thing to do. What ethical debate and deliberation can offer are ways of thinking about problems, ways of identifying the values that may be in conflict, and ways of systematically clarifying issues.

In this book, we base many of our discussions around cases, and we discuss the ethically relevant features in relation to the cases. In our discussions, we draw upon three standard approaches to ethical analysis. These involve looking at the consequences of different courses of action, looking at the duties or obligations of those making the decisions, and looking at the character and virtues of the decision-maker. In ethical terms, these three approaches are called consequentialism, deontology, and virtue ethics.

Consequentialism

As its name suggests, consequentialism is the view that it is the consequences of actions that determine their morality. This is an appealing view, as it links morality to the effects of our actions. Most of us intuitively consider the consequences of actions when we think about the goodness or badness of those actions. This is particularly so in medicine, where we rely upon the good consequences of our actions to help patients. Why is it good to remove an infected appendix? Because this restores the patient to health; the operation has beneficial consequences. It is belief in the good consequences of our actions that lies behind our therapeutic interventions.

The most famous consequentialist theory is utilitarianism, which links consequences with maximizing welfare or happiness. Many people are familiar with the utilitarian saying: 'the greatest good for the greatest number'. Utilitarians believe that the consequences of actions are morally important, so far as they affect the welfare or happiness of people. Actions that promote welfare are morally preferable to those that do not promote welfare. In addition, actions that maximize welfare are morally preferable to those that do not maximize welfare.

How does this work in practice? Utilitarianism requires working out which consequences matter and to whom. The welfare of each person affected by the action must be considered in the calculation, with each person counting for one, and no one counting for more than one (Hare 2001). So if we have an action, for example prescribing antibiotics for a woman with a urinary tract infection, there will be a good consequence for the patient in terms of her welfare, and we do not anticipate any ill consequences. The action seems morally worthy. Should we consider anyone else in the calculation? Probably not in normal circumstances, but if the woman had to be seen as an emergency in preference to another patient with severe back pain, or if there was a shortage of antibiotics, so that her treatment precluded treatment for a child with pneumonia, then we would have to include the harms to those other people in our calculation. It is in the practical details that utilitarianism and consequentialism become difficult. Utilitarianism requires assigning a value to each consequence. But how do you give a certain state of affairs a value? One approach is to focus on people's preferences or the satisfaction of their wants and desires. The utilitarian using this approach attempts to find out what people would prefer to do when they have a range of possible choices, takes account of how strongly they feel about their choices, and tries to ensure that as many preferences are fulfilled as possible. Despite the apparent simplicity of this approach, assigning a value to outcomes is notoriously difficult. How do we weigh up the value of a short life with cancer compared to a longer life in and out of the oncology unit for chemotherapy, or the uncertainty and risks of spinal surgery compared with the pain of a chronic disc prolapse?

Apart from these practical problems, consequentialism does not take account of the unintended consequences of actions, and yet we often believe that accidental outcomes should be judged differently from intended outcomes. If the woman prescribed with antibiotics has a severe anaphylactic reaction (despite no history of sensitivity to the drugs in question), this outcome harms her welfare. We do not however, judge the doctor to be morally blameworthy in the way that we would if he had set out deliberately to harm her.

Despite some of the difficulties, consequentialism plays an important role in our moral reflection. At many points in this text, we will delineate and take account of the outcomes of actions. However, we shall also consider other morally relevant factors, such as the duties of those involved, and their character and motives.

Deontological theories

Deontological theories hold that there are inherent or intrinsic features of acts that are morally significant, rather than their consequences. These theories are concerned with specifying duties in relation to acts that are either morally prohibited or required. Modern deontology is based upon the Kantian principle of unconditional respect for persons. This principle requires always treating others (and oneself) as ends in themselves, rather than as means to ends (Boyle 2001). Following this principle gives us duties not to deceive or coerce people, as this does not treat them as ends in themselves. If a GP enrols a patient in a drug trial without telling them about the payment that the GP receives for each enrolment, the patient might benefit from the drug and be none the wiser about the GP's financial arrangements. The consequences might be very satisfactory for both patient and GP. But a deontological analysis would maintain that the GP's action was wrong, because he deceived the patient, and used the patient's involvement in the trial to benefit himself.

Duty-based theories in health care often focus upon the duties and obligations that arise out of the specific circumstances in which we live and work. In this book, we will be concerned chiefly with duties that attach to the role of general practitioner. We will explore a number of these duties in some detail—duties to keep faith with those with whom one has agreements, to prevent harm and promote good, to respect the autonomous choices of others, to ensure that others receive their fair due, to be trustworthy. Out of these duties grow some specific rules and practices. The duty to obtain informed consent for medical treatment for example, is grounded in the principle that we should respect the autonomous choices of others. The duty to tell the truth and be honest in communication between doctors and patients is grounded in the obligation to avoid deception and to be trustworthy.

Just as consequentialist theories have problems, so too do duty-based theories. One difficulty is the problem of deciding on a course of action if duties seem to conflict. Based upon the principle of respect for persons, GPs should respect the autonomous choices of their patients. We have already alluded to some of the difficulties in knowing when a decision is autonomous. Apart from this, difficulties may arise if patients ask us to do something that breaches other duties. For example, the elderly man with cerebral secondaries in the example above did not want us to tell his daughter of his condition, but honouring his request involves deception towards his daughter on the GP's part. How should we weigh up obeying one duty that is in conflict with another?

Duties and consequences are morally important. Both of these approaches involve our original question: 'What is the right thing to do?' and offer answers that are justified by appeals to fundamental principles or to the consequences of actions. There is another way to approach our question, and this turns us away from judging actions, to looking at the characteristics and motivation of the person who is acting.

Virtue ethics

Virtue ethics directs our attention to particular qualities and character traits that are morally relevant. Our question about the right thing to do is answered by saying: 'The right thing to do is what a good person would do.' This approach is appealing for general practice because so much of general practice is grounded in the doctor–patient relationship, and the moral quality of the relationship depends very much upon the qualities that each person brings to it. Qualities like honesty, compassion, integrity, and justice are likely to support a good relationship, while deception, laziness, and greed will undermine the relationship. Virtue ethics relies upon identifying a series of virtues that are necessary for human flourishing, that is describing a set of characteristics that we accept as good for humans to live fulfilling lives (Oakley 2001). In health care, virtue theories link to the goals of medicine, so that beneficence is an important virtue, as are compassion and respect. Trying to do what a good GP would do in these circumstances can be a helpful action guide, particularly if we have been lucky enough to work with one or more GPs whom we admire for their wisdom in ethically challenging circumstances. We return to the question of the virtuous GP in the final chapter.

Conclusion

General practice shares various features with other branches of medicine, but the combination of features that occurs in general practice makes it unique. All of the features that we have mentioned in our discussions, the importance of the relationship and the comprehensive and continuing nature of care, lead to ethical complexity and raise ethical issues that are deserving of specific consideration. In our case discussions in the following chapters, we pick up on all three approaches to ethical analysis that we have discussed here. Sometimes, situations will seem to lend themselves more to one sort of reasoning than another. At other times, one or other perspective will provide an appropriate corrective to an unbalanced analysis. What is central to our interpretation of ethics in general practice is the relationship between doctor and patient. This is explored in depth in the following chapter.

References

Boyle, J. (2001). An absolute rule approach. In Kuhse, H. and Singer, P. (ed.) *A companion to bioethics*, pp. 72–9. Blackwell Publishers, Oxford.

Christie, R. and Hoffmaster, B. (1986). *Ethical issues in family medicine*. Oxford University Press, New York, NY.

Doyal, L. (1999). Ethico-legal dilemmas within general practice: moral indeterminacy and abstract morality. In Dowrick, C. and Frith, L. (ed.) *General practice and ethics: uncertainty and responsibility*. Routledge, London.

Hare, R. (2001). A utilitarian approach. In Kuhse, H. and Singer, P. (ed.) *A companion to bioethics*, pp. 80–5. Blackwell Publishers, Oxford.

McWhinney, I. (1997). *A textbook of family medicine* (2nd edn) Oxford University Press, New York, NY.

Oakley, J. (2001). A virtue ethics approach. In Kuhse, H. and Singer, P. (ed.) *A companion to bioethics*, pp. 86–97. Blackwell Publishers, Oxford.

Pellegrino, E. (1983). The healing relationship: the architectonics of clinical medicine. In Shelp, E. (ed.) *The clinical encounter: the moral fabric of the patient–physician relationship*. D. Reidel Publishing Company, Dordrecht.

Starfield, B. (1998). *Primary care: balancing health needs, services and technology*. Oxford University Press, New York, NY.

Further reading

Downie, R. S. and Calman, K. C. (1994). *Healthy respect: ethics in health care* (2nd edn) Oxford University Press, Oxford.

Doyal, L. (1999). Ethico-legal dilemmas within general practice: moral indeterminacy and abstract morality. In Dowrich, C. and Frith, L. (ed.) *General Practice and ethics: uncertainty and responsibility*. Routledge, London.

Chapter 2

Trust and the doctor–patient relationship

Introduction

Case 2.1

It is Dr Mira Shah's first day at work in the Pembroke Crescent Practice in Fetways. During morning surgery, the receptionist asks her if she can see an extra, a young child with a fever. Dr Shah agrees, and Mrs Barnes brings in her two-year-old son Trevor, saying that he has been very flat with a fever since last night. On examination, Trevor is drowsy and febrile, with marked neck stiffness and photophobia. Dr Shah makes a diagnosis of meningitis and arranges for urgent admission to the

Case 2.1 *(Cont.)*

nearest hospital, giving a dose of iv antibiotics as recommended by the paediatric registrar on duty. At lunchtime, she tells Dr Day (the long-standing principal in the practice) of Trevor's illness, later confirmed by the hospital as bacterial meningitis. He and the practice nurse who is in the room fall inexplicably silent, until finally Dr Day explains: Mrs Barnes is regarded as a difficult patient/mother by the practice, frequently requesting urgent appointments and home visits for apparently trivial illnesses in her children. If the receptionist had rung Dr Day, he would not have seen Trevor urgently. Thinking about the possible consequences of a delay in treatment is a sobering experience for Dr Day.

In this chapter we examine the doctor–patient relationship in general practice and ask, what kind of values are important in this relationship? The first part of the chapter explores trust, looking at moral reasons for patients to trust doctors, and doctors to trust patients. In the second part of the chapter, we look at the kind of issues that arise when there are problems in the relationship. The material in this chapter is closely linked to the contents of other chapters; there are specific cross-references to help you make these connections.

What is the doctor–patient relationship?

The meeting between patient and GP is at the centre of health care in general practice (McWhinney 1997). The consultation is the medium for people to access their GPs and through which GPs provide clinical care. Within the consultation, the nature and quality of the health care provided is largely dependent upon the nature and quality of the interaction. The term 'doctor–patient relationship' refers to this specific interaction, which may be characterized in various ethical, medical, and technical ways. Why is the relationship between doctor and patient so important, and why has it become one of the defining features of general practice?

It may be helpful if we think of the relationship as the substrate or foundation upon which care occurs. In a flourishing relationship, this foundation is strengthened over time and reinforced by positive interactions. This strong basis is then capable of supporting major events such as providing care through serious illnesses, or ongoing support for chronic ill health. These are instrumental benefits of the doctor–patient relationship: with a well-functioning relationship, it is easier for the GP to provide better health care, and outcomes may be improved. A lot of general practice research attempts to measure and define various aspects of the GP–patient relationship and relate these to outcomes such as patient satisfaction, compliance with treatment, patient recall of information, and resolution of symptoms (Stewart 1995; Winefield *et al.* 1995; Vick and Scott 1998; Howie *et al.* 1999; Little *et al.* 2001; Flocke *et al.* 2002).

Trying to define the instrumental benefits of the relationship may distract our attention away from another important issue—the intrinsic value of the relationship. By intrinsic value, we mean that the relationship is of value in itself, over and above any measurable improvements in health outcomes or greater patient satisfaction. Of course, there is a lot more to say here; not all relationships are rosy and, like any other relationship, the one between a GP and a patient may be harmful or destructive. The unstated premise is that particular kinds of relationships are of value, and it is part of the task of ethics to work out just what is valuable in a 'good' GP–patient relationship.

The importance of the relationship to general practice

In Chapter 1 we briefly discussed the central role of the GP–patient relationship, and reasons why it is considered so important. One of the main reasons for the centrality of the relationship is the ongoing commitment to individual persons, rather than to diseases or techniques, along with the holistic approach that this entails. Holistic care requires that GPs know their patients in a more thorough and robust way than for some other kinds of medical care. Finding out and using this information is part of a good relationship.

The continuing and open-ended nature of general practice provides the scope for relationships to evolve, in response to the changing needs and demands of both parties. GPs have to respond to any and all problems that patients present. This job is a lot easier if the GP can draw upon their store of personal information about the patient. In a good relationship there are established patterns of communication or behaviour, and each person knows more or less what to expect from the other. Drawing upon the capital of the relationship can help GPs to sort the urgency of symptoms; the onset of pain in a known stoical and infrequently attending patient will be taken far more seriously than a similar pain in a patient with a different pattern of physical symptoms and level of anxiety about health.

Finally, much of general practice is concerned with problems that do not sort into neat pathophysiological conditions. Often the diagnosis is uncertain, or the problem relates to psychosocial issues, or there is no 'medical' solution. In these cases, the GP herself is the therapeutic agent, and how well or ill the patient feels will depend upon the GP's skill at building the relationship. In cases when there may not be any specific medical action to take, the nature of the interaction and the relationship in which this is grounded assume relatively greater importance.

Of course, some of these features may be shared with other kinds of medical care, such as paediatrics or some branches of internal medicine, but no other speciality has embraced the doctor–patient relationship as a defining feature in the way that general practice has.

The importance of trust

Ethical interest in the doctor–patient relationship has focused upon defining particular features, in terms of rights and responsibilities, the character of the interaction, power issues, and decision-making. There are many different ways to classify the relationship. This is commonly done along a spectrum from consumerist to paternalistic.

These two extremes of the doctor–patient relationship are a useful way of drawing our attention to important ethical values in the relationship, such as acting for the patient's good, and respecting patients' autonomy. Beneficence and respect for patient autonomy are important ethical values, but on their own they do not exhaust the range of values which may occur in the relationship. (For further discussion of beneficence and patient autonomy, see Chapters 4 and 6.)

We believe that trust is a central and crucial ethical value in the GP–patient relationship. We take it for granted that patients should trust their doctors, although what this means exactly is not always clear. Whether doctors should trust patients is a question that is asked less often. Before looking at the ways that trust influences the relationship, we need to spend a little time analysing what we mean by trust.

Box 2.1 Consumerism and paternalism: the ethical extremes of the doctor–patient relationship

Consumerist

Consumerist relationships consider the patient as a client or consumer, and the doctor as a technical adviser. Patients/consumers have the right to have as much information as they need to make their own decisions about health care. The doctor's role is to provide the information to the patient, and then to help the patient to carry out their decision. Consumerist relationships are based upon the ethical value of respect for patient autonomy. The emphasis is upon patients making their own choices about what happens to them in terms of their health care.

Paternalistic

Paternalistic relationships are the opposite extreme. The patient is regarded as vulnerable and unable to make decisions, and the doctor is seen as the expert who knows what is best for the patient. The doctor has all of the power and makes the decisions; the patient is a passive recipient of care. Paternalistic relationships are based upon the ethical value of beneficence, or acting for the good of the patient. The emphasis is upon the duty of doctors to act in their patients' best interests.

When we call someone trustworthy, we are usually commending them in some way. When we invite someone to trust us, we are making a statement about our motives, and our honesty and reliability. Trust involves being optimistic about the person trusted in two main ways:

(a) Is the person competent to do what we are trusting them to do?

(b) Does the person bear goodwill towards us, so that they will respect our trust and do what we are expecting them to do (Jones 1996)?

Trust leads to vulnerability as when we trust another person we usually grant them quite a lot of discretionary powers, which of course may be used to help or harm the person trusting (Baier 1986). If we trust the neighbour to look after our house when we are on holiday, giving him the key gives him equally the power to harm us by stealing things, or to help us by feeding the cat.

If we stop to think about it, consciously trusting another person involves examining our beliefs about that person, and making a judgement about the reasons we have for those beliefs (Holton 1994). But often we trust or distrust without really thinking, so that our trust or distrust may reflect our prejudices rather than a calm and cool evaluation of specific reasons to trust. Trusting can be a risky business (the neighbour may steal our heirlooms), but trust is a fundamental ingredient in relationships ranging from the politely co-operative through to intimate partnerships. One important feature of trust is the way that we feel if we are let down. If we really trusted the neighbour, we will feel very betrayed if they have stolen our possessions. This is in contrast to the annoyance or disappointment we might feel if we are merely relying on someone. For example, although we rely on the plumber to fix our tap, we do not usually trust him to come on time. When he is late, we might be annoyed but we do not feel betrayed. Trust leads to 'a readiness to feel betrayal should it be disappointed' (Holton 1994, p. 67).

Trust in the doctor–patient relationship

What kinds of trust might occur in the relationship between GPs and their patients? We usually speak of patients trusting their doctors, and this can cover a number of areas. Patients' trust may relate to the competence or the goodwill or both of the GP. If we asked a patient about trusting their GP, they might say things like: "I trust him to work out what is wrong, and to know what to advise. I trust that he is up to date with medical information, and that if he doesn't know what is wrong, that he will refer me to someone else who does. I trust that he will behave professionally and not betray confidential material or try to take advantage of my situation. I trust that when he recommends a treatment, it is because he believes this is the best treatment for me, and not because he is doing a drug trial. I trust that he will provide medical care even if there is no cure for my illness." The list could continue for longer, but even this brief start makes us realize the almost endless content of the trust that a patient might have in their GP.

Trust in one area need not extend to trust in other areas. A patient may trust the goodwill of their GP, in terms of confidentiality, communication skills, and the like, but may not trust their competence in some clinical areas. The practice nurse, for example, may be a much quicker and gentler syringer of ears than the GP. Conversely, a GP may be trusted with straightforward clinical problems such as hypertension or arthritis, but not with sensitive personal information about depression or abuse. In terms of being trustworthy, it might not always be obvious what it is that the GP is being trusted to do, so that trust may be unwittingly betrayed.

Case 2.2

Ms Joanna Silks goes to see her GP, Dr John Bowler, because she has had recurrent headaches. Dr Bowler takes a history and examines Ms Silks, and comes to a provisional diagnosis of tension headaches exacerbated by a recent change of job. Ms Silks leaves the consultation dissatisfied. Her sister also had headaches and was referred for a CT scan of her head, and Ms Silks thinks she also should have a scan. She does not trust Dr Bowler's diagnosis because she thinks he is just trying to save money by not referring her.

Dr Bowler is unaware of Ms Silks' reasoning, and does not realize that she does not trust his diagnosis. If Dr Bowler is competent in formulating his diagnosis, then this distrust is probably unwarranted, but it will be hard for him to regain trust unless he finds out exactly what Ms Silks expects, and explains to her why her case is not the same as her sister's.

Should GPs trust patients? Ideally, doctors should trust patients in three areas:

(a) Motive: this is to do with trusting that patients are genuinely seeking medical care and share the aim of diagnosing and managing a health problem. A GP might distrust a patient's motives if she thinks the patient is acting for some other reason such as malice, or to obtain access to drugs of addiction, or sick certification.

(b) Testimony: this is to do with trusting that patients are telling the truth without too many exaggerations or omissions, for example that the pain was as severe as reported and not an exaggeration to obtain more time off work or stronger pain killers.

(c) Competence: this is to do with trusting that patients are competent, both in the general sense of understanding information, and in the practical sense of being able to cooperate with management (Rogers 2002).

Being trusted feels good: patients who are accepted at face value and whose histories are believed feel validated by this. Trust provides a moral boost, together with reassurance that they are right to have consulted the doctor. In contrast, seeing a doctor who does not believe the history or who thinks the patient is malingering is a very difficult experience. In Case 2.1 at the start of this chapter, Dr Shah's partner no longer trusted Mrs Barnes to know when to call for a doctor, and his lack of trust in her testimony and competence might have led to tragic consequences. Dr Shah had no reason to doubt Mrs Barnes' request for an urgent appointment, and her basic trust in patients knowing when they need an appointment may have saved Trevor's life.

The benefits of trust

There are important ethical reasons why trust is important in the doctor–patient relationship. A willingness to trust is ethically valuable because trusting another person involves treating that person as a moral agent. Trusting implies that the person trusted is capable of taking responsibility for their decisions (Horsburgh 1960). A GP who trusts her patient has taken the necessary ethical step of recognizing the patient as a person, rather than seeing her as a passive recipient of care. This recognition of the individuality and capacities of the patient is a necessary part of respect for autonomy. It is also a central part of the holistic philosophy of general practice, and recognized as important in developing the GP–patient relationship (May and Mead 1999). Withholding trust denies patients the opportunity to act as a responsible moral agents, or to make their own health care decisions.

Trust may be therapeutic, in the sense that trusting a person may increase their trustworthiness, by positively influencing the trusted person's behaviour. In this sense, trust is a kind of moral support, allowing the person who is trusted the chance to live up to expectations. This kind of trust may occur, for example, in a relationship between a GP and a person with an addiction disorder. Sometimes extending trust in this situation can provide the moral encouragement that the patient needs to make therapeutic progress. In this situation trust is both a practical and an ethical approach to constructively influencing behaviour. Trust in this situation can be risky, as the other person may not be able to live up to those expectations. Just as people may live up to expectations, they may also live down to them. Never trusting a person means that that person can never show that they have become trustworthy.

Trust offers a way of altering the power imbalance in the doctor–patient relationship. In most situations, it is the patient who lacks authority, recognized expertise, and medical agency. They are also the one who is ill, and they are often at a socio-economic disadvantage. By offering trust, the doctor can shift this balance of power. This can occur in a number of ways. Listening to patients and accepting their accounts of ill health demonstrates trust in their testimony; this is particularly important if the patient has confusing or unusual symptoms that may otherwise be dismissed. Trusting patients' motives is important, as the degree of trust is likely to influence the GP's response to the patient. Imagine a patient with a work-related back injury. If she is well known to the GP and trusted, her care will reflect this and her GP will provide moral as well as medical support in her rehabilitation. However an unknown patient may not be trusted in this way, losing both the moral and medical support. Similarly, patients who are trusted to be competent are given control over their treatment, for example working out their own insulin requirements. This is important in terms of creating the opportunities for patients to exercise autonomy, and to regain some sense of individual control which may have been compromised by being ill. On the other hand, if patients are distrusted by their GPs, the burden of that distrust is added to the original health problem, creating a reactive cycle of hostility and inhibiting good communication and clinical care.

As well as these ethical reasons, there are a number of obvious practical benefits if there are high levels of trust in the GP–patient relationship. Communication is easier, with less need to challenge or check up on statements, and less anxiety about what can be said, for both doctor and patient. With trust, it is easier to define the goals of the consultation. In trusting relationships, patients are able to accept the frequent uncertainty that accompanies diagnoses (or lack of diagnoses) in general practice. The presence of trust gives the GP some discretionary latitude, which is an advantage in an area as unpredictable as medicine. It is not always, or even often, possible to describe all of the potential outcomes or arrange plans to cover these contingencies, but in the presence of trust, both the GP and the patient can be sure that the other will exercise appropriate discretion. Thus a patient not specifically warned about a rare side-effect can be trusted to notify the GP should this occur, in turn trusting that he will welcome her observation and respond appropriately.

A relationship characterized by trust provides the flexibility to meet the variable demands of changes over time and in health status experienced by patients. Part of the problem with consumerist or paternalistic models of the doctor–patient relationship is that both parties are locked into a certain way of relating that may not suit changing circumstances.

Case 2.3

Mr Lincoln is a healthy 42-year-old who sees his GP, Dr Day, infrequently, usually to discuss his preventive care options for the extensive travelling that he does. His relationship with Dr Day, developed over a number of years, follows a consumerist pattern: he asks for the medical information and goes away to decide which precautions to take, taking into account other factors such as the kinds of places that he usually stays in, and his budget. If he decides to have a vaccination or take malaria prophylaxis, he rings the surgery and asks for a prescription to be arranged. This relationship suits Mr Lincoln as he likes to be well informed and make his own decisions.

However, Mr Lincoln becomes very unwell, with weakness, fatigue, weight loss, and night sweats. When Dr Day tells him of the tests that are necessary to reach a diagnosis, Mr Lincoln hears only the words 'possible malignancy' and becomes very frightened. He doesn't want to go away and do his own research and make his own decision. He wants Dr Day to be in control, trusting him to make the appropriate choices about investigations. Later, after the acute phase of the illness, he regains his confidence and takes more control over his treatment.

If Dr Day had insisted on following the usual pattern of their relationship, we would consider him quite unfeeling and unresponsive to Mr Lincoln's drastic change in circumstances. Patients and GPs in strictly consumerist relationships would have trouble dealing with new situations if they lacked the trust to relate in new ways. However, Mr Lincoln knew Dr Day well enough to trust him in this crisis, and on the basis of this trust, to follow whatever advice he gave. Patients who are in relationships based upon trust are able to share the decision-making responsibility, trusting the GP to know and act in their interests.

Similarly, a relationship locked into a paternalistic pattern may have difficulty accommodating a patient's growing expertise as, for example, she becomes used to handling her disease and develops her own management strategies. When circumstances change, previously satisfactory patterns of relating may no longer be suitable. The presence of trust creates a climate in which changes in the relationship can occur more easily than if trust is absent, easing the transition into new ways of relating. Across the spectrum of relationships, trust acts as a safety net.

One way of thinking about the role of trust in doctor–patient relationships is to identify what it is that makes some relationships unacceptable. Paternalistic relationships are problematic when the doctor assumes control over the relationship, irrespective of the wishes of the patient. We can think of this as an imbalance of trust: the dotor is demanding trust from the patient, trust in the medical view about what is wrong, and trust in the GP's competence at treating it. At the same time, the doctor is withholding any reciprocal trust in the patient's capacities, and not respecting her competence for making decisions or managing her illness. On the other hand, we can imagine paternalistic relationships in which the patient willingly (and justifiably) trusts the doctor to act in her best interests, and the doctor is proceeding because he knows that this is just what he is trusted to do. (See Chapter 4 for a full discussion of paternalism.)

Consumerist relationships seem to be an attempt to exclude trust. The doctor is not trusted for her opinions or to make decisions for the patient, and her obligation to provide information is seen as a contractual rather than moral obligation. In the absence of any trust, this is likely to lead to impersonal medical care. For consumerist relationships to work in a morally robust way, the patient has to be able to trust the information provided by the doctor, and the doctor has to trust the patient enough to provide the necessary information, and then leave them to make their own decision.

Problems with trust

Unfortunately, the presence of trust does not guarantee an ethical relationship. People make mistakes, and trust when they should not, or withhold trust from others who are trustworthy. Trust and distrust colour the way we see the other person, and, as in the case of Mrs Barnes and Trevor, can make it difficult to see past our habitual expectations. What are some ways to trust wisely?

First, we can look at the motives of the person who is being trusted, to see if there are any conflicts between their motives and the demands of trustworthiness. For example, if a GP is being paid generously by a pharmaceutical company to recruit patients into a drug trial, patients might question the trustworthiness of that GP if she encourages them to take part. Similarly, if a patient with an addiction problem is seeking treatment for an apparently painful condition, the GP may rightly question the trustworthiness of the patient's account. Patients do not have ways of finding out information about GPs' potentially conflicting motives. This creates an imperative for GPs to be honest about their motives, with their patients as well as themselves.

Next, we can examine our own reasons for thinking that the other person is or is not trustworthy. Prejudice and stereotyping can bias our views about the trustworthiness of others. This can work both ways in the GP–patient relationship. Patients' assumptions about general practice may prevent them from trusting the GP's motives. The withholding of antibiotics for viral illnesses, or X-rays for low back pain, for example may be interpreted as cost-saving rather than good medical care. GPs may make assumptions about the honesty or competence of patients based on unreflective generalizations rather than consciously weighing the reasons for trusting or not trusting in each case.

Trusting someone who is untrustworthy usually means that one person is being deceptive, potentially exploiting the person who is trusting. These are unwelcome ethical harms in themselves, but it is also worth looking at the consequences of misplaced trust in the doctor–patient relationship. For GPs, if a patient has been deceptive, there is the risk that the doctor's time and efforts are wasted or misplaced, for example trying to find an organic cause for a fictitious complaint. There is also the risk that the patient will come to harm, for example if a complaint of pain motivated by opiate addiction is taken on trust as 'genuine' pain, the patient is harmed through misdiagnosis and further access to opiates. Doctors often feel betrayed by addicted patients; this seems to reflect professional vulnerability, as not recognizing an addict can be seen as a professional failing. These harms from trusting untrustworthy patients are borne by the GP. In other cases however, the risks are borne by society rather than the individual doctor. For example, if a patient gains unjustified access to sickness benefits or compensation, it is the social welfare system rather than the doctor him or herself who has to pay the benefits.

For patients, the risks of trusting an untrustworthy doctor can be far more direct and personal. In extreme cases, misplaced trust can lead to death, either through incompetence or, very unusually, malice. Usually the consequences are not so drastic, but it is hard to measure the kind of harm that occurs when a doctor is untrustworthy due to incompetence or lack of goodwill. Patients cannot always judge competence, and doctors are often loathe to blow the whistle on their colleagues. This professional silence, as well as protecting untrustworthy doctors, may also foster a more general distrust of doctors. (See also Chapter 9.)

In summary, trust plays a crucial role, both moral and practical, in doctor–patient relationships. Relationships based on warranted trust may range from paternalistic to consumerist; in these cases it is the presence of reciprocal trust that makes the relationships morally acceptable. Trust is easy to withhold, but when patients are not trusted, this can hamper good medical care as well as impose extra burdens upon patients. These observations about trust imply that there is an obligation for GPs to consciously, and demonstrably, be trustworthy, and to trust patients unless there are justifiable reasons for not trusting.

So far we have discussed the doctor–patient relationship in fairly abstract terms, emphasizing the possible benefits. What happens when things go wrong in the relationship?

Difficult relationships

A well-functioning doctor–patient relationship tends to drop out of sight, with straightforward communication, productive negotiations, and apparently effortless decision-making. In reality, the situation can be much more difficult. Relationships may become difficult if there are tensions between intimacy and professionalism, if there are relationships that extend beyond the consultation, or if unacceptable gifts are offered. Sexual attractions between doctors and patients raise ethical issues, as do relationships with patients who are very dependent or needy.

The balance between intimacy and professionalism

One of the most difficult areas concerns the limits and boundaries of the relationship between GP and patient. We have outlined an ideal relationship of mutual trust and respect, but is it realistic to expect this kind of relationship to remain strictly limited to the consulting room? How should caring and involved GPs reach the appropriate balance between intimacy and professionalism with their patients? Within the consultation, GPs hold much more personal knowledge about their patients than the other way around. Sharing some personal information with patients can be a way of strengthening the relationship and building trust, but this is a matter for individual judgement. Some patients are the sort of people that we are usually friends with, so that it seems natural to tell them something about personal events. Some patients like to think of their GP as a person with a life and interests outside the consultation room, and appreciate being able to assemble a more complete picture of their GP. Other patients prefer a strictly professional relationship.

The doctor–patient relationship may reach beyond the consulting room in a number of ways. Patients may have relationships with their GP in other contexts, such as in community work, or on committees. Sometimes even acknowledging patients outside the consultation can breach confidentiality, unless the greeting is initiated by the patient. It seems unreasonable to avoid any social interaction with people who are also patients, but at the same time the GP must try to distinguish between any social roles and their role as GP. This might require discussion with the other person, to clarify how best to balance professionalism within a developing friendship. Not discussing health problems outside the consultation is a common sense way of protecting the boundary, as well maintaining confidentiality. At times it can be hard to maintain the boundaries, especially when different relationships require different roles. A patient who is in a more casual role in one context may find the greater formality of the doctor–patient relationship difficult to adjust to, as may the GP involved. Problems in one relationship may spill over into other unrelated areas, leading to questions about when the doctor–patient relationship may be considered over.

Case 2.4

Miss Little has a longstanding relationship with her GP, Dr Oliver Whittaker. Miss Little and Dr Whittaker are members of the same community arts committee, which meets frequently. Miss Little has a chronic illness, for which she also sees a complementary therapist. The therapist advises a course of prescribed medication, available only through a GP. Dr Whittaker and his partner, Dr Bowler, have decided on a policy of not providing this treatment as it is not considered medically effective and is also very expensive. This refusal eventually leads to Miss Little moving off the practice list.

However, Dr Whittaker has ongoing contact with Miss Little through their community arts work. In this context, Miss Little is hostile and angry with Dr Whittaker, and indicates to other members of the committee that she has been badly treated by the Westminster Surgery. This creates a problem for Dr Whittaker. Should he continue to maintain the tenor of the doctor–patient relationship even though Miss Little is no longer a patient, or should he respond as he would to any person he is finding difficult to work with on the committee?

There are some options open to Dr Whittaker in this situation. Miss Little's medical information is confidential, so he cannot counter the charges with his own account of what has happened. Dr Whittaker can attempt to discuss the issue with Miss Little and ask her to separate the issues related to her medical care from their current work on the committee. If this is not successful, he is no longer morally obliged to treat Miss Little with the consideration that he would give to a patient. Dr Whittaker should be free to interact with Miss Little simply as a difficult committee member.

Information disclosed within the GP–patient relationship can have an impact upon the GP's personal life. For example, within the consultation a GP may become aware that a female patient is involved in an extra-marital affair. If this patient is also a close friend of the GP's wife, it can be hard for the GP to separate the professional from the personal. How should he react to the patient/friend of his wife in social situations, and should he withhold the information if his wife voices suspicion about her friend's marriage? The GP's obligation to the patient includes confidentiality, but he may consider asking her to change GPs if he feels that her ongoing care is causing tensions within his own intimate relationships. (See Chapter 3 for a full discussion of confidentiality.)

Gift-giving

Gift-giving within the doctor–patient relationship is another area with ethical dimensions. The giving of gifts can range from natural expressions of goodwill through to attempts at bribery. Many patients offer small gifts to their GPs, such as home-made jam or articles of clothing for the GP's newly arrived baby. Refusing these gifts can seem heartless and unnecessary. Problems may arise however when the gifts are inappropriately generous or seem to be given for an ulterior motive. A patient might give an expensive gift in an attempt to secure preferential treatment or speedy referral. Some gifts may not be directly related to medical care, but may be attempts to gain an advantage in business dealings with the practice. The GMC offers advice on receiving gifts when there is a possible conflict of interest, stating that doctors should not put themselves in a position in which their judgement about a patient's care could be questioned with regard to any party from whom they have received gifts (GMC 2001). Given that doctors have a duty to make the care of the patient their first concern, there is no theoretical advantage in giving a gift to secure better care! There is no hard and fast definition of what constitutes a 'significant' gift. One common rule of thumb is to refuse any gift unless you would be willing for information about that gift to be made public. Many practices avoid the potential difficulties associated with gifts from patients by having a practice policy covering issues such as acceptable limits of gifts, and the distribution of gifts either to charitable institutions (local hospital or old people's home) or to practice staff (Champ *et al.* 1995). Any policy on gifts should be publicized to patients. This kind of approach is preferable to an opportunistic approach in which only unwanted gifts are passed on.

Is it always unethical to accept significant gifts? Perhaps the most difficult situation arises when a patient wills a significant gift to their GP. An elderly person with no close relatives might prefer to leave particular items such as books to a well-known and liked GP rather than to a distant relative or to a charity. Accepting a gift in this circumstance will not affect the GP's judgement with regard to the patient, as the patient is dead. Ethically speaking, accepting the gift might be a way of respecting and honouring that patient's memory. Decisions about accepting gifts willed by patients need to be made by the individual involved, bearing in mind possible accusations of unprofessionalism or trial by media. What might actually be an ethical response in terms of accepting the books may be distorted or mis-represented to the GP's detriment. The issue of gifts from the pharmaceutical industry is covered in Chapter 9.

Sex and the GP–patient relationship

Almost any relationship offers opportunities for sexual involvement, and the GP–patient relationship is no exception. What are the ethical considerations here? The main concern is that the professional relationship provides GPs with access to patients in vulnerable and intimate situations, and that the relative power of GPs over their patients can make it very difficult for patients to refuse sexual advances. Sexual contacts in this situation are for the benefit of the doctor, betraying the obligation of doctors to act in the patient's best interests, and also likely to compromise the health care that the patient receives. In ethical terms, this is a betrayal of trust, violating the duties to act in the patient's best interests and to do no harm. Sexual exploitation of patients is regarded as one of the most serious professional offences and is severely punished both by the General Medical Council and in the courts.

Does this mean that it can never be ethical to have a sexual relationship with a person who is also a patient (White *et al.* 1994)? If there is mutual attraction, the respective roles of doctor and patient may seem irrelevant except as a perhaps unusual method of introduction. The main ethical consideration must always be the interests of the patient, and avoiding any situation that exploits the patient or compromises their care.

The doctor–patient relationship may lead to transference on the part of the patient, making it almost impossible to ever consider the patient as an equal party to any relationship. Patients who have received psychiatric care or counselling are particularly vulnerable to sexual and emotional exploitation by their treating doctor. Is it an abuse of medical power if a GP first meets a person as a patient, and then pursues the relationship outside the context of medical care? It is impossible to give an answer that covers all possible situations, but in the initial stages of any relationship that starts like this, the roles of GP and prospective partner are blurred. This is the case even if the person has not been a patient for some time, or if the length of formal GP–patient relationship was brief.

As well as possible harms to patients. GPs who enter such relationships are also potentially vulnerable as they may be open to charges of sexual harassment. In addition, patients may lose trust in a GP who is known to engage in relationships with their patients. Overcoming these ethical barriers would require extra-ordinary care, indicating that relationships with ex-patients should in general be avoided.

Situations of one-sided attraction require sensitive handling.

Case 2.5

Dr Mira Shah has not been in Fetways long before she realizes that one of her patients, John Monford, has become infatuated with her. Mira and John meet socially through a shared interest in a local National Trust property, and on these occasions John makes comments about Mira's attractiveness. Dr Shah gains real pleasure from her National Trust activities, so she does not want to discontinue her involvement. At the same time, she does not want to do anything to encourage Mr Monford or to foster intimacy, but she does not feel that she has grounds to ask him to leave her list. One day, Mr Monford consults with a number of problems, one of which requires rectal examination.

In this situation, there are a number of considerations. The first is to provide the patient with the care he needs, and the second is to respect Dr Shah's right to practice without feeling forced into uncomfortable personal situations. Referring the patient to her partner Dr Day for his rectal examination is one way of avoiding unwanted physical intimacy, while continuing herself with less intimate care. This may be possible without directly raising the subject of the patient's feelings for Dr Shah. In general, early discussions with colleagues or partners reduce the burden upon the GP and provide support in finding an acceptable solution. What if the situation is reversed so that it is the GP who is attracted to the patient who remains unaware of the attraction or does not welcome it? Proceeding with intimate examinations in this context betrays the patient's trust that the interaction is solely to meet their medical needs.

Most discussions of sex and the doctor–patient relationship focus upon the vulnerability and/or exploitation of patients. However research from Canada suggests that sexual harassment of female GPs by male patients is also a problem (Phillips and Schneider 1993). In their survey well over two-thirds of the respondents reported some kind of harassment ranging from suggestive looks and sexual remarks through to rape. The power relations in this situation are complex: the doctor has the power and authority of her position as a medical practitioner, but at the same time is female in a society in which some men use their strength and power to sexually intimidate women. General practice can create very vulnerable situations in which GPs are alone with patients, sometimes in the patient's home. In addition, the duty of care means that female GPs cannot refuse to see male patients for whom they are responsible, therefore cannot completely avoid any situations of risk. We believe that sexual harassment by patients is a betrayal of the medical relationship, and that women GPs are entitled to take any necessary actions to be safe in their work. These might include a practice policy on not working alone in the practice, immediate reporting of any offences, and support from other partners in allocating home visits.

Needy or dependent patients

Many GPs experience difficulties in their relationships with patients who have needs that are hard to meet in the medical context. These might be patients with medically unexplained symptoms, or with minor mental illnesses, or addiction disorders. Patients with these problems often leave the GP feeling helpless and inadequate, as whatever they suggest does not seem to alleviate the patient's problems. What is the ethical response of the GP in this situation? Issues of trust, patient autonomy, and acting in the patient's best interests can be hard to sort out. What does a patient with unexplained symptoms trust the GP to do, and in what ways should the GP trust the patient? A basic ethical requirement here is to trust that the patient is in distress and is making a genuine request for help. This can be difficult in the face of unacknowledged psychological illness, or denial about addictions. It may not be possible in the initial stages of the relationship to trust the patient's testimony or competence, but trust that at some level, the request for help is genuine seems to be fundamental to building a therapeutic relationship. Once the GP has accepted that the patient wants help with a problem, she can then consider other ethical aspects, such as the potential to benefit or harm the patient, and how the patient's autonomy can be respected.

Case 2.6

Julian Servante is 35-year-old male patient who is well known to Dr Carter. He has multiple problems including headaches, irritable bowel syndrome, joint pains, and tiredness. His symptoms increase at times of stress such as moving house and increased pressure at work. In the past Dr Carter has performed many investigations including blood tests, abdominal X-rays, and a CT scan of the head. All investigations have been normal, but despite this, Mr Servante remains anxious and feeling unwell, and makes frequent requests for referrals, especially to a neurologist and to a gastroenterologist.

We can consider Dr Carter's possible actions in terms of harms and benefits to the patient. Investigations can exclude serious or urgent pathology, and may alleviate some of the patient's anxiety. On the other hand, investigations can also increase anxiety and a focus on physical symptoms (Salmon *et al.* 1999). Some investigations are potentially harmful, such as endoscopy or exposure to radiation, and all run the risk of false positive or negative results. Referrals to specialists usually entail further investigations. There are also the patient's wishes to consider, and what he is trusting the GP to do. Patients who feel let down by the medical system may have very little trust, requiring consummate communication skills on the part of the GP to explain their therapeutic approach.

A further complication relates to diagnostic and therapeutic uncertainty. Whilst there is general agreement that patients with these kind of problems are difficult to work with, there is disagreement about the terminology ('medically unexplained symptoms', 'somatizing disorders' 'heart sink', 'fat-file syndrome', etc.) and the nature of the problem (Butler and Evans 1999). It seems likely that there is a constellation of as yet poorly understood problems, requiring different approaches. In this situation, building trust through open and honest communication ensures that the patient receives the therapeutic benefits of an ongoing doctor–patient relationship. This does not mean that the GP must offer an open-ended response; part of the therapeutic response may require setting limits and providing regular but limited access. What is ethically required are respectful and honest responses about what the GP can do, acknowledging the limits of medical approaches, but offering ongoing care despite the limitations. Recognizing the value of building a relationship may alleviate some of the pressure that GPs feel to 'do something', sparing both patients and the public purse the cost of unfruitful investigations and referrals.

Collusive relationships

As we have discussed above, the doctor–patient relationship can be an important therapeutic tool, providing the foundation for health care. However, sometimes the relationship can seem take on a life of its own, and both GP and patient may become locked into a relationship which meets some needs, but not perhaps the needs of health care. Collusion can develop when the GP acts from a desire to please the patient or preserve the relationship at any cost, rather than acting for the medical good of the patient. Collusion may initially seem harmless, such as agreeing with a patient's medically bizarre account of their symptoms. The situation becomes more difficult if patients request investigations or therapies which are not, according to current standards of evidence, medically effective and/or warranted in the circumstances (see also Chapter 4). Giving in to these kind of requests may seem an attractive course of action as pleasing people is far easier than refusing them, and there may be harm to the relationship if the refusal is seen as unwarranted by the patient. Collusion may also occur if the doctor is frightened of the patient, either physically or in terms of complaints or litigation. Balanced against these reasons are the ethical requirements to act for the medical good of the patient and to be trustworthy rather than deceptive. Agreeing to provide medically unwarranted services is generally dishonest and undermines the growth of morally decent trust.

Conclusion

In this chapter we have proposed a perhaps idealistic doctor–patient relationship based upon trust. The doctor–patient relationship is the backbone of general practice, and trust is one of the necessary elements for that relationship to flourish. Trusting patients will not necessarily transform all GP–patient relationships into rosy ones, but consciously thinking about trust can help to flesh out some of the moral responsibilities that both doctors and patients have towards each other, making it easier to consider other important ethical issues that occur in practice.

References

Baier, A. (1986). Trust and antitrust. *Ethics* **96**, 231–60.

Butler, C. C. and Evans, M. (1999). The heartsink patient revisited. *British Journal of General Practice* **49**, 230–3.

Champ, R., Haslam, D., and Lewis, W. (1995). A patient who keeps giving expensive gifts. *Practitioner* **239**, 695–8.

Flocke, S. A., Miller, W. L., and Crabtree, B. F. (2002). Relationships between physician practice style, patient satisfaction, and attributes of primary care. *Journal of Family Practice* **51**, 835–40.

General Medical Council (2001). *Good medical practice*, Paragraph 55 http://www.gmc-uk.org

Holton, R. (1994). Deciding to trust, coming to believe. *Australasian Journal of Philosophy* **72**, 63–76.

Horsburgh, H. (1960). The ethics of trust. *The Philosophical Quarterly* **10**, 343–54.

Howie, J. G., Heaney, D. J., Maxwell, M., Walker, J. J., Freeman, G. K., and Rai, H. (1999). Quality at general practice consultations: cross sectional survey. *British Medical Journal* **319**, 738–43.

Jones, K. (1996). Trust as an affective attitude. *Ethics* **107**, 4–25.

Little, P., Everitt, H., Williamson, I., Warner, G., Moore, M., Gould, C. *et al.* (2001). Observational study of effect of patient centredness and positive approach on outcomes of general practice consultations. *British Medical Journal* **323**, 908–11.

May, C. and Mead, N. (1999). Patient-centredness: a history. In Dowrick, C. and Frith, L. (ed.) *General practice and ethics: uncertainty and responsibility*, pp. 91–106. Routledge, London and New York, NY.

McWhinney, I. (1997). *A textbook of family medicine*, (2nd edn). Oxford University Press, New York, NY.

Phillips, S. and Schneider, M. (1993). Sexual harassment of female doctors by patients. *New England Journal of Medicine* **329**, 1936–9.

Rogers, W. A. (2002). Is there a moral duty to trust patients? *Journal of Medical Ethics* **28**, 77–80.

Salmon, P., Peters, S., and Stanley, I. (1999). Patients' perceptions of medical explanations for somatization disorders: qualitative analysis. *British Medical Journal* **318**, 372–5.

Stewart, M. A. (1995). Effective physician–patient communication and health outcomes: a review. *Canadian Medical Association Journal* **152**, 1423–33.

Vick, S. and Scott, A. (1998). Agency in health care. Examining patients' preferences for attributes of the doctor–patient relationship. *Journal of Health Economics* **17**, 587–605.

White, G. E., Coverdale, J. A., and Thomson, A. N. (1994). Can one be a good doctor and have a sexual relationship with one's patient? *Family Practice* **11**, 389–93.

Winefield, H. R., Murrell, T. G., and Clifford, J. (1995). Process and outcomes in general practice consultations: problems in defining high quality care. *Social Science and Medicine* **41**, 969–75.

Further reading

Baier, A. (1995). *Moral prejudices: essays on ethics.* Harvard University Press, Cambridge, MA. See especially Chapters 6–9 on trust.

Cassell, E. J. (1991). *The nature of suffering and the goals of medicine.* Oxford University Press, New York, NY. See especially Chapter 5: The mysterious relationship between doctor and patient pp. 138–57.

General Medical Council (2001). *Good medical practice.* General Medical Council, London. *http://www.gmc-uk.org/standards/default.htm*

O'Neill, O. (2002). *Autonomy and trust in bioethics.* Cambridge University Press, Cambridge.

Rogers, W. A. (2002). Is there a moral duty for doctors to trust patients? *Journal of Medical Ethics* **28**, 77–80.

Chapter 3

Confidentiality in general practice

Introduction

Case 3.1

Joanna Silks has been Dr Bowler's patient, on and off, for many years. She has anxiety and depression that are related to childhood sexual abuse and a difficult relationship within her marriage. She and Dr Bowler have had a rather unusual relationship: periodically, Joanna gets angry with him and decides she doesn't want him to be her GP any more. She then attempts to seek out another GP, but has never actually removed herself from his list.

This time, Joanna came with a range of symptoms that Dr Bowler thought were related to her ongoing distress, and he thought she might have irritable bowel syndrome. Despite his endeavours to convince her otherwise, she insisted on a referral to a surgeon. Dr Bowler was generally happy to comply with patient wishes in this kind of situation, but he thought the surgeon needed to know something

Case 3.1 *(Cont.)*

of her background history. Accordingly, he included a note in his referral letter about her anxiety and depression.

At the Westminster Surgery, practice referral letters are sent with the patient in a sealed envelope. Joanna opened the letter and read it. It was about her, so Dr Bowler didn't have any problems with her doing that. Joanna, however, didn't like being described as a patient with an 'emotional disorder'. She came back to see Dr Bowler and said: "No, I don't want this in the letter, but I still want the referral." Dr Bowler rewrote the letter.

Dr Bowler didn't feel all that comfortable about leaving out what he thought was important background for the surgeon. On the basis of his history, examination, and investigations he didn't believe that the referral was an appropriate referral anyway but, as he said to his partner, Oliver, the next day: "If a patient requests and insists on a referral, it is very hard not to refer." And he felt that the surgeon would have wanted to know. He thought it would make the surgeon's job much easier; it would have allowed him perhaps to ask questions in a way that would have explored some of the issues more effectively. Knowing Joanna, Dr Bowler suspected that if the surgeon had asked for the background, she would have denied it. He thought the surgeon probably would have worked it out anyhow, but he would have handled it better if he had access to something of what Dr Bowler knew about Joanna.

Maintaining patient confidentiality has a long and venerable history in medical practice. Many GPs will be familiar with the promise of confidentiality found in the Hippocratic oath:

> Whatever, in connection with my professional practice, or not in connection with it, I see or learn, in the life of man, which ought not to be spoken abroad, I will not divulge, as reckoning that all such should be kept secret.

As an obligation on medical practitioners, it is also enshrined in more recent codes of ethics, including the General Medical Council guidance:

> Patients have a right to expect that information about them will be held in confidence by their doctors. Confidentiality is central to trust between doctors and patients. Without assurances about confidentiality, patients may be reluctant to give doctors the information they need in order to provide good care. If you are asked to provide information about patients you should:
>
> a. Seek patients' consent to disclosure of information wherever possible, whether or not you judge that patients can be identified from the disclosure.
>
> b. Anonymise data where unidentifiable data will serve the purpose.
>
> c. Keep disclosures to the minimum necessary.

GMC 2000

What, exactly, is confidentiality? Why is it important? When, if ever, may or must a doctor breach confidentiality? This chapter explores these questions.

What is confidentiality?

Confidentiality is a duty: it is something doctors have a moral and, often, legal obligation to maintain for their patients. In general, the duty of confidentiality requires that doctors keep secret the information they are given by a patient and/or which they discover or learn about patients through their professional interactions. Patients can expect that:

(a) All information they disclose to the doctor will not be passed on to a third party without the express consent of the patient.

(b) The doctor will take reasonable steps to protect the information collected from patients from access by third parties (Beauchamp and Childress 2001).

It is important to note a couple of things about this definition. First, patients can freely waive the right to confidentiality. If a patient authorizes release of information, it is not a violation of the duty of confidentiality to provide it to those to whom the patient has authorized the release. Had Joanna agreed to the disclosure to the surgeon of all aspects of her history, Dr Bowler could have passed that information on without a second thought.

Secondly, 'information' needs to be interpreted fairly broadly. It includes not only what the patient says, the findings on examination, results of tests and procedures, diagnoses and outcomes of treatment, but includes what the patient may unconsciously convey (for example, their emotional state), and the fact that the person has been a patient at all (Hamblin 1992, p. 423).

Finally, the doctor's obligation to keep confidences relates not only to what he or she may consciously pass on to others about patients; it includes accidental and unwitting releases of information about patients. For example, leaving patient records open on the reception desk where visitors to the practice may see them, discussing a patient in an identifiable way with a colleague in a lift (Ubel 1995), and taking a call from or about a patient while another person is with you may all be violations of the rule of confidentiality. These sorts of violations of confidentiality are particularly important in small, rural communities, where it is quite likely that people can piece together the identity of a patient from bits of information. Some of these inadvertent violations are unavoidable, but others are merely careless. Just because a doctor did not intend for sensitive information to reach the ears of others doesn't make it acceptable. 'I didn't think of it' is not a moral argument.

One of the most significant issues for confidentiality is the sharing of information about patients that goes on within health teams. In a world in which the one-to-one relationship between doctor and patient is often complicated by group practices, specialization, team management, quality assurance mechanisms and the like, it can be very difficult to uphold a promise of absolute confidentiality. It was his awareness of these practices that prompted Siegler in 1982 to suggest that confidentiality was a 'decrepit concept' that had past its prime.

Siegler and others may have been correct to be pessimistic about the future of confidentiality. Certainly, in the twenty years that have passed since his article, violations of confidentiality of the type he described have become increasingly common. However, the ubiquity of such breaches does not necessarily mean that they are justified. We still need to examine the ethical reasons for confidentiality, and the situations in which breaches may be ethically acceptable.

Why is confidentiality important?

On a daily basis, we are surrounded by situations in which information about people is not kept confidential. The recent glut of reality TV shows bears witness to the extent to which some people are willing to live with little or no privacy. How can we justify a rule of confidentiality for general practitioners? What makes not keeping a confidence wrong?

Confidentiality is important for a number of reasons. Some of these reasons relate to what confidentiality can achieve for individual patients and the broader society. Other reasons focus on what confidentiality expresses—respect for patient autonomy and a promise kept with society. How these reasons function to justify maintaining of confidentiality is important not just as a matter of philosophical interest, but particularly to help us work out what to do when we think breaches of confidentiality are justified.

Confidentiality offers benefits for individual patients, both in terms of their likely usage of health services and the quality of care they may receive. Some patients may not seek medical care unless they are assured of confidentiality. For example, adolescent girls may be less likely to seek contraceptive advice if they know their parents may be told. People diagnosed with HIV may present later in their illness if there is mandatory reporting. Once in the consulting room, such patients will not be completely open and honest with their doctor unless they know that what is said in that room will be kept secret. There is a real limit to how well a doctor can diagnose, treat, and care if patients provide only a partial account of themselves and their illnesses. The promise of confidentiality has an important bearing on the relationship of trust between individual doctors and patients.

Confidentiality in the doctor–patient relationship also has benefits beyond those that accrue to individual patients. Some people argue that an environment in which confidentiality is taken for granted is essential to provide the climate of trust and confidence that we need for any health care to be provided. Put another way, it would lead to poor outcomes for everyone if we did not have rules of confidentiality in medicine. Not only might individual patients suffer because of the reasons already outlined, but also the community would lose trust in the medical profession and in medical care. Doctors would not be able to do their jobs properly because they would never be sure that the information on which they were basing their decisions was accurate.

We do not necessarily know, in real life, whether confidentiality rules always increase the quality and outcomes of medical care. If you could show that the patient, their family, or the community in general, would be better off if confidentiality were breached, then it might be acceptable not to keep a confidence. We will look at some reasons for breaching confidentiality below, but for now it sufficient to note that, regardless of how good or poor these utilitarian arguments for confidentiality are, there are other, deontologically-based arguments that also support a rule of confidentiality for doctors.

The first of these deontological arguments is that confidentiality is important because it expresses respect for patients' autonomy. We explore the notion of respect for autonomy in detail in Chapter 5.

Here we merely note that respecting others' autonomy includes acknowledging that patients have aspects of their lives that they should be able to keep secret if they choose. It also means taking care to ensure that patients are not observed, touched, or intruded upon without their consent. Some of us are more concerned about our privacy than others but, in our individualistic society, the right to be able to choose who has access to information about us is generally accorded a very high value. And doctors, by virtue of their professional work, often have access to highly personal, sometimes shameful and embarrassing, information, information that many people do not want revealed to a wider audience. When patients provide doctors with information, that information continues to belong to the patient and he or she can expect that the doctor will not pass on information about them to unauthorized others.

A final way to justify the rule of confidentiality is to see it as deriving from the obligation that all doctors have to keep faith with their community. The key idea here is the notion of keeping promises and commitments. How is keeping a promise or a commitment related to keeping information about patients confidential? After all, we don't make an explicit promise to each and every patient we see. However, there is a *social* expectation that doctors will keep information about patients secret. In a sense, when you become a doctor, you promise the community that you will keep the information patients give you confidential. Having made that promise, you 'no longer start from scratch in weighing the moral factors of a situation' (Bok 1983). You have already committed yourself to respect the confidentiality of the information you are given, so that divulging that information to other people is like breaking a promise. This type of argument helps to explain why we think it acceptable to tell others what our next door neighbour paid for his house, or our views about the quality of work of the local plumber, even though it is unacceptable to chat about patients with a friend (Rhodes 2001, pp. 498–9).

We have set out four related reasons for why confidentiality is important. While these reasons offer powerful arguments for why we should not break the rule of confidentiality, it is very important to recognize that there are some circumstances in which it is permissible, and sometimes even necessary, on either moral or legal grounds, to breach confidentiality. The next section explores situations in which confidentiality can be a problem.

Cases in which confidentiality can be a problem

The primary obligation that general practitioners have to maintain confidentiality is simply stated. It is much harder to define those circumstances under which it is acceptable to break a confidence. In general, breaches of confidentiality fall into one or more of the following groups:

(a) Situations in which we are unsure whether patients are in a position to decide for themselves.

(b) Situations in which it seems to be in the best interests of the *patient* to break the rule of confidentiality.

(c) Situations in which it seems to be in the best interests of *others* to break the rule of confidentiality.

When patients may not be able to decide for themselves

Some of the most difficult cases are those in which the general practitioner is concerned that the patient is not really able to make a competent choice. For example, consider Dr McDonald's position here.

Case 3.2

Lucy, a 13-year-old girl, comes to see her GP, Dr Fiona McDonald. Dr McDonald has known Lucy from childhood, and she has cared for all members of her family. Lucy has never attended on her own before and seems quite nervous. Eventually she says that she would like to go on the pill, to make her periods regular. After some discussion, Lucy explains that she has a 15-year-old boyfriend and that they are planning to have sex, but that she is very worried about the possibility of pregnancy. She has read about contraception in magazines and thinks that she would prefer the certainty and 'lack of fuss' of the pill compared with barrier methods. Lucy is worried that her mother, whom she describes as 'overprotective', would be thrown into a panic if she learnt about Lucy's intentions. She asks Dr McDonald for a prescription, and for assurance that she will not reveal her request to anyone.

Dr McDonald is probably not sure what to do. On the one hand, she wants to protect Lucy's confidence; on the other, she is tempted to contact Lucy's parents. One of the reasons Dr McDonald is unsure of the right thing to do is because the foundations on which the promise of confidentiality is built seem to be in doubt here. First, Dr McDonald may not be sure that Lucy is really able to function as an autonomous decision-maker. (See Chapter 7 for a full discussion of Gillick competence.) Is she really old enough, at 13, to make this decision on her own? And, having made the decision, is she mature enough to carry the burden of concealment? Confidentiality may be justified by the principle of respect for autonomy, but when we have doubts about the autonomy of the patient, that justification can seem rather weak. For this reason, it *may* be permissible for Dr McDonald to tell Lucy's parents.

Adolescent contraception and pregnancies are not the only situations in which general practitioners can face questions about confidentiality and competence. Drug and alcohol abuse, psychiatric illness, and mental disability can all raise questions about the capacity of a patient to make an autonomous decision.

When breaching confidentiality may be in the patient's best interests

Even if Dr McDonald has no concerns about Lucy's competence or maturity, she may be tempted to breach confidentiality for a second reason. Dr McDonald may wonder whether keeping this kind of information secret is in Lucy's best interests. What if Lucy were pregnant and seeking an abortion? Dr McDonald might worry that Lucy would need support from an adult in that situation, or she may feel that no one should have to face such decisions alone.

Dr McDonald's reasons are similar to the reasons Dr Bowler might have offered for breaching confidentiality. When Dr Bowler included a comment about Joanna's psychosocial history in his referral letter, he was doing what he thought would be in her best interests. He naturally included in the letter those aspects of Joanna's medical history that he considered relevant for the management of her current condition. He believed that Joanna's psychosocial history was important; he probably also knew, given her concern not to be described as someone with an 'emotional disorder', that it was unlikely Joanna would tell the surgeon herself about her anxiety and depression.

A lot turns, in these two cases, on how confident the general practitioners can be that their judgement of the patients' best interests is the correct one. The interpretation of patients' best interests is a complex moral issue which we discuss in detail in the next two chapters. Here we note only that, while it is true that more openness about the patient's condition can often have significant benefits for patients—through more accurate diagnosis, more appropriate treatment, or better support in distressing situations—it is also true that patients do not always see such things in the same light as their doctors do. For example, Dr McDonald may think Lucy will benefit from the support of her family; Lucy may know that the 'support' will consist mainly of criticism and complaints about her selfish conduct. Dr Bowler's frequent contact with people in psychological distress may lead him to understate the stigmatizing effect of mental illness for Joanna. There is a conflict here between a justification for confidentiality that is based on privacy, autonomy, and promise keeping, and one that is based on the best interests of the patient. This is one of the central issues for medical ethics, and we return to it again in Chapters 4 and 5.

When breaching confidentiality may be in the best interests of others

The final group of problems for confidentiality relates to situations in which GPs think that other people may be harmed or, at least, not helped if they do not break a confidence. Case 3.3 provides an example of just such an ethical dilemma.

Case 3.3

One evening Margaret Brown presents to the surgery with an obvious case of delirium tremens due to acute alcohol withdrawal. Despite being a well-known patient, this is the first time that Dr McDonald is aware that Margaret has an alcohol dependency problem, and that she usually drinks half a bottle of vodka per day while working as a registered childminder caring for children in her own home. The doctor advises admission but Margaret refuses as she has children booked in for the next day.

Dr McDonald is concerned that Margaret is intoxicated whilst caring for children, and that the children may be at risk of harm because of this. Margaret promises to stop drinking.

Case 3.3 *(Cont.)*

Over the next few months Margaret appears to be refraining from alcohol. In the meantime, Dr McDonald has attempted to clarify the ethical and legal situation. Her Medical Defence Union has advised her that if the patient has given her word that she is not drinking, then Dr McDonald has no right to breach confidentiality on the grounds of possible danger to the children in her care. The opinion of the defence union is that the GMC would consider striking off Dr McDonald if she breached confidentiality and the patient complained.

David Grainger, one of Dr McDonald's partner, feels very strongly that Dr McDonald should notify social services, using the 'What would the papers say?' argument. What would the papers say if there was a fire and a child was injured as a result of the childminder's intoxication and Dr McDonald had not acted despite her knowledge of the danger?

Social services, contacted by telephone with a general inquiry, were not interested in the situation as their resources are stretched to the limit dealing with actual cases of child abuse: 'Children are looked after by drunk parents all the time and we don't interfere.'

A few months later Margaret is obviously drinking again. Dr McDonald urges her to stop work. Margaret says that she will contact the childminder's registration authority and inform them that she is no longer active. However, suspension of work is voluntary, and childminders can recommence work whenever they wish without giving a reason for their break and without any re-registration processes.

Dr McDonald contacts a friend in social services and explains the nature of the problem. She is concerned that the voluntary nature of the arrangement may not hold, and that Margaret may start caring for children again at any time. The social worker advises calling the registration authority.

Dr McDonald calls the registration authority and asks to know the status of Margaret's registration. The authority wants to know why. Dr McDonald replies that she cannot give the reason. After some further conversation, the registration authority ask whether it will be satisfactory if they ask for Margaret to return her registration certificate, which means that she will require a full health care check prior to become registered again. Dr McDonald says, 'Yes'.

This dilemma caused much anxiety for Dr McDonald who felt very strongly that if she did not act, children were potentially at risk. She felt that there was no one to consult over a problem of this kind, and that the attitude of the defence union was less than helpful.

In contrast to other situation in which GPs do have a duty to notify of possible danger to the public (e.g. bus driver with epilepsy), there are no procedures for notifying about problems with childminders, despite their occupational responsibilities towards the children they care for. Given the vulnerability of children, and the fact that the children themselves are not likely to notice anything amiss in the behaviour of their carer, what should Dr McDonald's responsibilities be in this case?

It is worth noting, at the beginning of our discussion of this case, that it takes place in a particular legal and social context. There are a small number of situations in which GPs are required, by law, to provide information about patients to third parties, usually to a clearly specified organization such as the police or the health department. Although the precise requirements will vary from country to country, in general GPs are required to pass on information about patients, without their consent if necessary, when:

(a) Reporting notifiable diseases, including sexually transmitted diseases.

(b) Notifying births and deaths (including underlying cause of death).

(c) There are concerns about a patient's fitness to be granted a driver's licence.

(d) When child abuse is suspected or confirmed.

Some of these situations are relatively straightforward. The decision to breach or not breach confidentiality often becomes a non-decision when the law *requires* such breaches. For example, death certificates are legally required to be completed honestly and fully, to the best of the doctor's knowledge and belief (GMC 2000). Sometimes, if the cause of death is thought to be potentially stigmatizing such as suicide or HIV/AIDS, the relatives of the deceased may request that the cause of death is not written on the certificate. Such requests may be very understandable to the GP, but there are other factors to consider. Death certificates are important epidemiological data; their usefulness depends upon their accuracy. The public duty to provide accurate information outweighs the individual interests of the bereaved. In addition, inaccurate death certificates may be used for fraudulent insurance claims.

Completing the death certificate is a required and acceptable breach of patient confidentiality. Information may also be legitimately supplied to a coroner or procurator fiscal in connection with an inquest, or in accordance with the Access to Health Records Act 1990, for example to an insurance company. Apart from these exceptions, doctors have a duty to maintain confidentiality about their patients, even after death, unless authorized to do otherwise by the legal executors of the patient's estate.

The fact that the law does require GPs to break confidences in some situations is of some relevance to the ethical issues at hand here. Waller puts it well when he notes that, in situations in which passing on information to others is mandated, 'the legislature has, presumably, there done the business of balancing competing interests; medical confidentiality has been outweighed by the public interest in the administration of justice, or the community's general health, or the prevention of serious crime' (Waller 1993, p. 198).

Waller's point is that, in these circumstances, we could, if we were inclined to follow the argument through, justify breaches of confidentiality because other people's interests outweigh individuals' concerns to protect their privacy. The 'other' interests relate to two groups. First, there are interests that can be linked to identifiable individuals. For example, GPs may become aware of inherited diseases, such as Huntington's disease, that are carried by some members of a family and of which other members of the family are unaware. They may be torn between wanting to respect a patient's desire for secrecy and realizing that other family members should have access to relevant information before they make important decisions about careers, marriage, and child-bearing.

In the *Tarasoff* case, which came before the Californian Supreme Court in 1976, the failure by a psychologist to breach confidentiality had tragic consequences for an identifiable individual. The *Tarasoff* case concerned a university student who confided to the psychologist treating him at a university counselling service that he intended to kill his girl friend, Tatiana Tarasoff. The young woman was clearly identifiable. The psychologist was concerned enough to attempt to have the student committed for psychiatric evaluation. His efforts were unsuccessful, and the patient was released from temporary custody police and ended his therapy. Neither the psychologist, nor the police, made any attempt to warn Tatiana, or her family, that her life might be in danger. Two months later, the student killed Tatiana. Her family sued the psychologist and the University for damages and the Supreme Court of California held that both were liable, on the grounds that the psychologist had a duty to attempt to prevent harm to an identifiable individual and that there was clear evidence that Tatiana was in grave danger.

The second group of interests are those which can not necessarily be linked to identifiable people. In these cases, we may not be able to tie the benefits to be gained (or the harms to be prevented) by breaching confidentiality to recognizable individuals. It may be, rather, that we think the breach is warranted on the grounds of benefits to society as a whole or to particular groups in society. The rationale for mandatory reporting of sexually transmitted diseases to the health department or informing road traffic authorities that a patient is not fit to drive falls into this category. In the second case, particularly, it is almost impossible to identify precisely the people who might be harmed if an unfit driver continued to drive.

Such situations are interesting from a public policy point of view, and they are similar in type to the ethical dilemma that Dr McDonald faces. However, they do not raise the acute problems that Dr McDonald experiences. Dr McDonald's moral dilemma is complicated because her attempts to create some certainty for herself have, so far, been ineffective.

Dr McDonald's unsuccessful search for legal and regulatory clarity is probably not an isolated incident. These cases are immensely difficult and the law does not always offer GPs clear guidance on what they should do (Hamblin 1992; Waller 1993). In recent times, the courts have had to consider a number of cases in which a breach of confidentiality, on grounds of the public interest, was the central issue. Fortunately or unfortunately, the courts have arrived at conclusions that suggest only that 'there is very little certainty as to how a court will determine the operation of the public interest exception in any given case' (Hamblin 1992, p. 430). In this environment, what can Dr McDonald do, and why should she do it?

As she thinks about these issues, it may be helpful for Dr McDonald to attempt to clarify the *size* and the *risk* of harm to the children in Margaret's care. She may also wish to think about the extent to which whatever she can do will actually prevent the harm from occurring. Put another way, Dr McDonald might ask herself: 'Is there a *substantial* risk of *serious avoidable* harm to others in this situation?' (Beauchamp and Childress 2001, pp. 308–9). Let's look at each of the issues identified in this question in turn.

First, what is the size or seriousness of the harm that might befall others? Is someone's life in danger? Or, is it rather that a third party will merely experience minor, self-limiting harm if the doctor does not breach confidentiality? In general, the more serious the harms that may arise if a GP does not intervene, the greater the likelihood that the GP's intervention can be regarded as ethically acceptable. In this case, the harms that might befall these children are variable. At one end of the spectrum, Margaret's drinking may mean only that the children do not get fed on time, or that they spend all day watching television. If these were the extent of the harms likely to befall the children in Margaret's care, Dr McDonald would probably have little justification for interfering. After all, as the social services office implies, many children are not adequately cared for, but society rarely intervenes to rescue them. In this case, though, there are other, far more serious, consequences that may arise if Margaret drinks to excess while caring for children. Dr McDonald's colleague has already raised the possibility of a fire; one could equally imagine a child running on to a road, injuring himself in a fall, or drowning in a bath. Any of these events would have serious consequences for the children.

The seriousness of the harm is not the only issue to take into account. The second component to our question relates to the size of the risk or the probability that the harm will occur. How likely is it that the harm will actually eventuate? Again, the higher the probability or risk of harm, the greater the obligation on the GP to intervene. In Tatiana Tarasoff's case, the psychologist was concerned enough about the likelihood that his patient would act on his stated intention that he sought to have him detained. He considered that the risk of harm to Tatiana was quite high. This will not always be the case and there will be situations in which the GP may realize that the risk of harm to others is actually relatively low. Dr McDonald's dilemma falls somewhere in between and she may require more information to assess the risks accurately. For example, she may need to assess how likely it is that Margaret will take up work again. Obviously, the risk of harm to children evaporates when Margaret is not childminding. But, will Dr McDonald be in a position to know if Margaret goes back to work? Beyond these considerations, some people might argue that the risk of calamitous events here is actually quite low, and perhaps not all that much higher than the background level of risk for all children.

Finally, Dr McDonald will need to consider the extent to which whatever she chooses or is able to do can somehow change things for the children Margaret cares for. Dr McDonald's actions so far have had some impact. However, it is still possible that, despite her intervention, Margaret may continue to do informal, unregistered childminding. If Dr McDonald decides that breaching confidentiality by informing the registration authority is not really going to change things, then she ought to reconsider whether informing the authority at all has been worthwhile. Alternatively, she may need to think about other actions she can take that are more likely to protect the children from harm. For example, she could take the drastic step of trying to inform parents that their childminder was drinking heavily while caring for their children.

When Dr McDonald has considered these issues, she still has to weigh the harms and/or benefits for the children against the need to respect Margaret's confidences and to act in ways that are in Margaret's best interests. This balancing, and the decisions that follow from it, will always be difficult.

Conclusion

In this chapter, we have explored the ethical issues that arise from the obligation to respect confidences. Although confidentiality is not an absolute duty, in most cases, breaching confidentiality requires a heavy burden of proof. Reaching an ethically acceptable decision will often hinge, in large part, on weighing the relative merits of patients' best interests and the duty to respect the autonomy of patients. The philosophical underpinnings of these concepts are discussed in the next two chapters.

References

Beauchamp, T. L. and Childress, J. F. (2001). *Principles of biomedical ethics*, (5th edn), pp. 303–12. Oxford University Press, New York, NY.

Bok, S. (1983). The limits of confidentiality. *Hastings Center Report* **13**, 24–31.

General Medical Council (2000). *Guidance on good practice. Confidentiality*. London: General Medical Council. *http://www.gmc-uk.org/ global_sections/search_frameset.htm.*

Hamblin, J. (1992). Confidentiality, public interest and the health professional's duty of care. *Australian Health Review* **15**, 422–34.

Rhodes, R. (2001). Understanding the trusted doctor and constructing a theory of bioethics. *Theoretical Medicine and Bioethics* **22**, 493–504.

Siegler, M. (1982). Confidentiality in medicine: a decrepit concept. *New England Journal of Medicine* **307**, 1518–21.

Ubel, P. A., Zell, M. M., Miller, D. J., Fischer, G. S., Peters-Stefani, D., and Arnold, R. M. (1995). Elevator talk: observational study of inappropriate comments in a public space. *American Journal of Medicine* **99**, 190–4.

Waller, L. (1993). Secrets revealed: the limits of medical confidence. *Journal of Contemporary Health Law and Policy* **9**, 183–210.

Further reading

Beauchamp, T. L. and Childress, J. F. (2001). *Principles of biomedical ethics* (5th edn), pp. 303–12. Oxford University Press, New York, NY.

General Medical Council (2000). *Confidentiality: protecting and providing information.* General Medical Council, London. *http://www.gmc-uk.org/ standards/default.htm*

Siegler, M. (1982). Confidentiality in medicine: a decrepit concept. *New England Journal of Medicine* **307**, 1518–21.

Chapter 4

Beneficence, or does the doctor know best?

Introduction

Case 4.1

Sibyl Price presents to Dr Jeremy Chu with tiredness. On examination, Dr Chu detects enlarged cervical and axillary nodes. The nodes are rubbery rather than tender. Dr Chu's first impression is that this could be leukaemia or lymphoma, with viral infection as a secondary diagnosis. He arranges blood tests without explaining to Mrs Price the likely causes of her illness or the specific investigations.

If we asked Dr Chu what he is doing, he may well reply that he is acting in the best interests of his patient. What does this mean? In our example, Dr Chu might say that he is medically trained and has expertise in formulating symptoms and signs into a working diagnosis, and then confirming this with relevant investigations. Performing the blood tests is a way of checking the accuracy of his working diagnosis, and it is his job to know which tests to perform and how to interpret the results. As the patient has no training in medicine, there is no point in discussing with her which tests to do.

Dr Chu might also say that Mrs Price is feeling unwell, she is anxious as well as tired, and that it is not fair to burden her with possible diagnoses until the clinical situation is clearer. He might say that it is part of the doctor's responsibilities to keep silent about all the possible diagnoses, especially potentially serious ones, and that the patient expects him to sort out the problem and then tell the patient, rather than involving the patient in the fear and uncertainty of tentative diagnoses.

He might also say that part of the therapeutic power of medicine lies in this kind of power and responsibility, and that the patient feels better if her care is provided by a doctor who takes charge. The patient's confidence may be undermined if the doctor does not act in a directive way that indicates he is in control of the situation. Later in the chapter we shall analyse these justifications in detail, but first we shall examine the ethical obligation which underlies the idea of acting in the best interests of the patient.

The principle of beneficence

The principle of beneficence imposes a duty upon doctors to act always for the good of their patients. This is the very heart of morality—one of the ways we judge the goodness or badness of an action is by asking the question: 'Are we trying to help or harm?' We can think of this in two ways, in terms of underlying motives, and in terms of the actual effects or consequences of our actions. In medicine it is difficult to be certain that our actions will always lead to good outcomes; we cannot guarantee this in advance. However, we can examine our motives, and ask whether our action is motivated by the aim to benefit the patient. In general, medical practice is considered inherently beneficent, as it promises assistance to the sick or injured, aiming to mitigate the harm of ill health. (See also Chapter 10 on the virtuous practitioner.)

As an ethical principle, beneficence is central to most codes of professional ethics. Under the duties of a doctor listed by the GMC, the first is: 'make the care of your patient your first concern' (GMC 2001). Similarly, the Hippocratic Oath says that: 'I will prescribe regimen for the good of my patients according to my ability and my judgement and never do harm to anyone' and 'In every house where I come I will enter only for the good of my patients.'

The Hippocratic Oath picks out two important aspects of beneficence. The first is to do with using medical expertise to help rather than harm the patient. The medical knowledge that doctors have is specialized and generally unavailable to patients. As this knowledge could be used either to help or harm patients, accepting the obligation of beneficence harnesses that power for patients' good and limits the potential for harm.

The second part of the quote: 'I will enter only for the good of my patient' refers to the privileged position accorded to doctors. Doctors collect private information about patients, and have extensive physical access to their patients. Both of these privileges could be abused, for example by gossiping about a patient's intimate affairs, or performing unnecessary breast examinations. Being aware of the patient's good and acting beneficently will help to ensure that these privileges are respected.

As the expression of a moral ideal, acting for the benefit of others is straightforward; difficulties arise however, when we try to determine what kind of obligations should guide our actions in general practice. In general, there are three kinds of problems when we try to work out what it means in practice to act for the good of patients. The first is working out what we mean by the good of the patient, the second is treading the fine line between beneficence and paternalism, and the third concerns questions about what is medically good.

Acting in the patient's best interests

In some situations, it is very straightforward to say what acting in the patient's best interests might be. If we think back to Trevor's case in Chapter 2, it was in his interests to be treated immediately for meningitis. Similarly, a person with severe chest pain has their interests served by prompt investigation to confirm or exclude myocardial infarction. For many consultations in general practice, there is an obvious health problem for which it is in the patient's best interests to receive advice or treatment.

Yet often things are not so straightforward, and this can be especially the case in general practice where there can be conflicts between the health interests of a person and other important interests that the person might have. There may be tensions between a person's health interests and their employment interests.

Case 4.2

Barry Black is an apprentice plumber who works for a fairly unsympathetic boss. He presents to Dr Shah with a badly bruised and sprained right wrist. The injury occurred when a piece of equipment broke while ditch digging. Dr Shah arranges for an X-ray to exclude fracture, and then the practice nurse straps the wrist. Dr Shah advises two weeks rest, followed by physiotherapy. Mr Black is reluctant to be signed off for this long, as he cannot afford the drop in income, and he knows that his boss will be angry if this is recorded as a work-related injury.

Barry's interest in maintaining his income and staying on the right side of his boss is in direct conflict with his medical interests.

The person with chest pain may be a single woman who cares for her daughter with Down's syndrome, and who does not wish to go to hospital for investigations or admission because this will leave her daughter with no carer. This would also force her to face up to the issue of who will care for her daughter when she can no longer do this.

These kind of conflicts are common in general practice, because general practice takes place within the community and GPs are constantly faced with the reality and importance of their patients' interests over and above any immediate health problems. In secondary and tertiary care, the health problem can be so urgent or overwhelming that the patient's interests have shrunk to coincide with their health interests. If the woman with chest pain has a heart attack, all of her interests rely upon successful treatment for the heart attack. But such urgent situations are rare in general practice, leaving GPs with the sometimes difficult task of negotiating the place of health interests for each patient that they see.

Sometimes it is hard for doctors to appreciate the other interests that patients have; medical training tends to foster powerful normative views about health and illness, so that doctors may feel very strongly about what the right thing to do is, with regard to health. This can lead to absurdity when carried to extremes.

Case 4.3

Mrs Stirling is a fit 85-year-old woman. She has some minor arthritis in her hands, for which she takes anti-inflammatories. When attending the Gordon Road Practice for a repeat prescription, Dr Grainger urged Mrs Stirling to have her cholesterol checked. Her cholesterol level was found to be slightly elevated, and Dr Grainger advised Mrs Stirling to cut down on her dairy products. Her sole dairy intake was a nightly mug of a malted milk drink, which she duly sacrificed for the sake of her cholesterol level.

Mrs Stirling was grateful to Dr Grainger for identifying this problem and alerting her to the dangers of drinking milk.

In this case, Dr Grainger used a narrow medical view of the patient's interests, understood solely in terms of serum lipid levels. On the basis of this, he prescribed changes in behaviour with no discussion of the actual risks for Mrs Stirling of continuing her nightly mug of milk, or the effect of this sacrifice upon her sleep patterns or overall enjoyment in life. General practice prides itself on taking a holistic view of patients; if this is to be taken seriously, GPs must take a wide rather than a narrow view of patients' interests when they consider their obligations to act beneficently.

Beneficence and paternalism

The duty to act beneficently applies to all doctors, but as we have said, the scope of patients' interests can vary by specialty and circumstances. In general practice, patients may present with a wide range of physical, mental, and social problems, so that to respond competently and comprehensively, GPs must use a broad understanding of best interests (Christie and Hoffmaster 1986). At times, beneficence takes the form of taking charge of the patient, leading us into the sometimes tricky region where morally justifiable beneficence may slip over into morally questionable paternalism.

What is paternalism, and why is it morally questionable?

Box 4.1 Paternalism

Paternalism involves acting for the good of another person in the way that a parent might act for the good of their child. There is an assumption that the person acting paternalistically is wiser, more knowledgeable, or more experienced than the person they act for, and this justifies taking charge. In medicine, we assume that doctors are more expert than patients, and that this can justify making decisions on patients' behalf. Some patients may expect or welcome doctors taking charge, but there are dangers if doctors assume that this is what patients want.

There are two kinds of paternalism.

1 Strong paternalism is acting for the good of the patient, even if this involves overriding the patient's wishes. This might happen if the GP admits an elderly patient to hospital even though she does not want to go.

2 Weak paternalism is acting for the good of the patient without acting against the expressed wishes of the patient (Sherwin 1992). This is like Case 4.1 at the start of this chapter.

The difference between paternalism and beneficence hinges upon the way that decisions occur, the extent to which the patient contributes to the decisions, and the attitude of the doctor.

Strong paternalism involves intentionally overriding patients' wishes, either openly or through deception. In general, these kinds of actions are morally unacceptable, because overriding patients' wishes denies patients the chance to make their own decisions, or in ethical terms, to act autonomously. This kind of paternalism should be rare, limited to situations in which there does not appear to be any other way of managing a situation, and in which the person is in danger of serious harm if the doctor does not act. There is further discussion of overriding autonomy in Chapter 6.

Weaker forms of paternalism are commoner in practice. These include assuming that the patient is not capable of understanding medical information, or deciding 'not to worry' the person with information because the doctor thinks that this may be burdensome. It is the assumptions that are paternalistic; the GP's intentions are to benefit the patient, but the assumption is that the GP knows how to do this without finding out what the patient would like. In the example at the beginning of the chapter, Dr Chu's decision not to discuss the reasons for the tests was paternalistic because he did not offer Mrs Price the chance to receive more information, or to decline particular tests. Instead he assumed the responsibility for knowing what wais best for the patient in the circumstances.

Paternalistic attitudes can be hard to pin down. These can be conveyed through language in phrases such as: 'You don't need to worry about this', or in condescending or overbearing behaviour (Downie and Calman 1994). The crucial point here seems to be that although the doctor may be acting for the good of the patient in terms of medically appropriate actions, there is no element of consent and the patient is not respected as a person who is capable of participating in decisions.

Justifications for paternalism

Dr Chu offered three familiar justifications for paternalism (Sherwin 1992).

Box 4.2 Proposed justifications for paternalism

1 The vulnerability of the sick: ill people are not in a fit state to make decisions, so that it better for doctors, who are unaffected by the illness, to make the decisions.

2 Medical expertise: doctors are the experts, so this makes them the right ones to make decisions for patients.

3 Medical confidence and the placebo effect: unless doctors are paternalistic, they will lose the healing power associated with patients having faith in their doctors.

In the following section we examine whether these justifications hold up in general practice.

The vulnerability of the sick

Are general practice patients too ill to discuss relevant information or make decisions? In some cases, for example unconscious patients, this is the case, and of course the GP should take responsibility for making decisions in that patient's best interests. Other forms of illness, even quite minor illness, can make a person feel fearful, tired, less capable, or not wanting to be bothered with decisions, and this may be accompanied by a desire to be cared for. This however, does not always translate into a desire for a paternalistic GP.

It may be helpful to identify two separate activities here. The first is to do with giving information and the second is to do with making decisions. These are often run together, but either information and/or inclusion in decision-making may be withheld by doctors for paternalistic reasons.

Patients who feel ill may not want to be faced with medical decisions, but they may welcome information and explanations about their situation. Of course, judgement must come into this, and part of the skill of general practice lies knowing the patient and knowing how much information they usually prefer. Paternalism creeps in when there is a unilateral decision by the GP that the patient does not need to know, or would be better off not knowing.

What if the patient is faced with a serious diagnosis? Are they still able to take in information and make important decisions? Serious diagnoses can be devastating, accompanied by fear, grief, and misery. This can impair a person's immediate capacity for decision-making. It would be naive to assume that a person can be given a diagnosis of lymphoma or breast cancer and then immediately be able to make important decisions. But usually there is no need for this kind of speed. Most medical decisions are not urgent; there is time to face the diagnosis, and talk about the patient's beliefs and wishes. This is particularly the case in general practice which offers the opportunity for patients to return after an initial diagnosis, to provide more information and to discuss the options.

The desire to spare patients uncertainty and fear can lead to paternalism. However, a paternalistic approach in this situation blocks the opportunity to discover the nature of the fears, and to sort out with the patient which fears are justified and to deal appropriately with those that are not. Ethically, it is preferable to discuss the patient's fears, so that a perhaps overwhelming fear of the unknown becomes replaced with fear of something more circumscribed and manageable. This approach supports the patient's capacity for decision-making, so that the patient is helped to participate in decision-making and there is no need for paternalism.

In many general practice consultations, patients are not ill. Chronic disease management, vaccinations, cervical smears or blood pressure checks, sick notes, and follow-up consultations all involve patients who are very much themselves, rather than feeling ill or fearful. This means that it is relatively rare in general practice that paternalism can be justified by appeals to the patient's vulnerability.

Medical expertise

The second justification for paternalism is that medical decision-making requires the medical expertise (scientific or technical knowledge) that is acquired through medical education. As doctors are the ones with this expertise, they should decide for patients. The assumption here is that medical decisions are mainly scientific/technical in nature. However, many of the decisions that occur in general practice are not like this. For example, if a patient consults with lateral epi-condylitis (tennis elbow), the issue might be whether or not to have surgery or conservative treatment. The patient needs access to some technical information in order to make a decision, but the decision itself is not technical as it cannot properly be answered on purely technical grounds. The answer depends on the values the patient puts upon various factors such as their dissatisfaction with present therapy, the need to remain at work, their inclination to take risks, or the waiting lists for different therapies. Of course there are situations in which doctors do know best in a straightforward sense, for example what kind of operation to perform once a decision to proceed with surgery has been reached, but situations with a single technical solution are the exception rather than the rule in general practice.

One way of thinking about these issues is in terms of domains of expertise. This approach recognizes that most decisions in general practice require the expertise of both patient and GP. Medical expertise is important, in interpreting symptoms, developing and confirming diagnoses, and suggesting options for management. The patient needs this expertise to understand their problem and to decide about management. But medical expertise alone is not enough to reach an optimal decision; the patient also has expertise that she brings to the consultation. She is the one who knows how the problem is affecting her and how serious it is. She is also the expert as far as knowing what kind of management options will be acceptable or possible for her. Thinking about both the patient's and the GP's expertise in an explicit way helps to make sure that they both have the best possible understanding of the patient's interests and how these can be furthered. The two domains of expertise are complementary, and both are necessary for a holistic understanding of the patient's interests (Rogers 1999).

Medical confidence and the placebo effect

A third justification for paternalism revolves around the idea that it is important for doctors to act confidently, as faith in the doctor is good for patients. If the patient believes that the doctor is right in their diagnosis and treatment, this belief contributes to the success of the treatment. The mechanism for this is unclear, but is attributed in part to the placebo effect. Two studies from general practice seem to demonstrate the beneficial effects of medical confidence. In the studies, one group of patients received a directive or positive style of consultation, and these patients were more satisfied, and some had significantly swifter symptom resolution than patients who received a negative or non-directive style of consultation (Thomas 1987; Savage and Armstrong 1990). A belief in need for medical confidence (and so harnessing of the placebo effect) is based on the assumption that the disclosure of uncertainty is a bad thing for patients, and that uncertainty decreases doctors' effectiveness as healers (Katz 1984).

Do patients really wish for certainty when they see a GP, or is it GPs who feel uncomfortable admitting or explaining or tolerating uncertainty? Not knowing a definite diagnosis may make doctors feel inadequate, and perhaps it is natural to counter this by giving the patient something definite, such as a prescription. Doctors may feel very uncomfortable doing nothing, because they think that the patient wants them to do something (Katz 1984; Christie and Hoffmaster 1986). In the past this has led to the widespread use of placebos, such as 'tonics' or 'cough bottles'. Perhaps the prescription of antibiotics for viral infections also falls into this category. If these are prescribed with sufficient authority and confidence, the patient may well feel better due to the placebo effect. This course of action can be attractive as the patient feels better, and the doctor also feels better as she has responded to a request for help in a positive way. The down side lies in the deception to the patient, and the fostering of expectations in patients for further prescriptions.

Is there any way of harnessing the placebo effect without deception or using prescriptions? Can we keep the therapeutic power of the doctor–patient relationship without being paternalistic? This is where trust plays a role: honesty about uncertainty may build trust and help to transfer the power of the placebo effect from the prescription to the doctor herself (Katz 1984). The GP can use the existing trust within the relationship to 'ask for credit', for example to explain that even though she is not certain of a diagnosis, serious problems have been ruled out, and the problem will almost certainly get better on its own. This kind of approach may be as powerful as a physical placebo.

What is the medical good?—the role of evidence-based medicine

If doctors are to act for the good of their patients, it is important that they know which treatments are effective and which are not. This is one of the main aims of evidence-based medicine (EBM), which attempts to ground health care in interventions that have been shown to be effective. At first glance, this aim fits in very well with ideas about acting in the patient's best interests, as it is surely in their interests to receive effective rather than ineffective or harmful treatments. Is using EBM a practical way of assisting GPs to act beneficently? There are some features about general practice that mean that using EBM (or evidence-based guidelines) to inform decision-making can be difficult, especially if GPs take an holistic approach to patient's interests (Rogers 2002).

Much of the evidence for EBM comes from randomized controlled trials, in which the trial population is restricted to a relatively homogeneous group with a single disease. In general practice, the population may be far more varied (with regard to age, gender, or ethnicity) than the research population, so that it is not clear whether the findings are applicable. More significantly, co-morbidities are common in general practice, yet people with co-morbidities are excluded from most research (Watt 2002).

EBM reviews provide statistical estimates about the effectiveness of treatments in trials. Other important factors which feed into general practice decisions include the preferences of the patient, the GP's knowledge of this particular patient, or information about the local availability of services. Knowledge about effectiveness on its own is not usually enough to reach a conclusion, as we need information about the goals of the patient before it makes sense to ask whether a particular treatment is an effective way of reaching those goals. EBM can lead to an excessive focus on the scientific basis of medicine, which may be inappropriate for general practice where personal and contextual features are an important part of practice (Jacobson *et al.* 1997).

However, EBM reviews are an important way of keeping up to date, and if there is relevant information about the effectiveness of treatments, this should be used in patient care. GPs describe various sources for their expertise, including professional experience, reading journals, personal experience, continuing medical education programmes, and discussion with colleagues (Rogers 1999). The balance between EBM and these other sources of expertise is something to be weighed up for each patient.

In practice, clinical guidelines are the working face of EBM. Evidence-based guidelines are developed using the principles of EBM, providing guidance for particular clinical scenarios. Many of these guidelines are quite paternalistic. Guidelines produced by National Institute for Clinical Excellence (NICE), or Scottish Inter-collegiate Guidelines Network tend to define a single management path without offering the opportunity for patients to choose amongst alternatives. There is a sort of shift here, instead of the GP being the medical expert, the guideline is now the expert who tells both the patient and the GP what to do. Rogers (2002) has analysed the ethical issues raised by guidelines use in general practice.

The limits of beneficence

Acting in the patient's best interests is a moral imperative for doctors, but at times this imperative comes into conflict with other considerations. These kinds of conflicts may be difficult to identify, and can cause significant unease. In the following sections we discuss some examples of the limits of beneficence (see also Chapter 6).

Patient-driven constraints

When consultations are patient-initiated, we trust that the patient is motivated by their health interests. By and large this is the case; patients come to see GPs because they have a health problem, and GPs are able to use their skills in addressing the problem. Conflicts may arise when the patient's aims diverge from the GP's, away from the course of action that seems indicated by considerations of health.

Case 4.4

Mrs Duke is a patient in her late sixties, who is an infrequent attendee at the Gordon Road Practice. One day she presented to Dr McDonald with abdominal distension and anorexia. On examination, Dr McDonald found a large mass

---

Case 4.4 *(Cont.)*

and ascites. Dr McDonald thought that the most likely diagnosis was ovarian cancer. She explained this to Mrs Duke and advised that some investigations would help to confirm the diagnosis and then it would be possible to work out what, if any, treatment would be recommended. Mrs Duke refused to have any investigations or to see a specialist for further assessment. She eventually died several months later.

In this case, Mrs Duke came to see Dr McDonald for a diagnosis, and then chose to decline further treatment, despite the explanations and encouragement of Dr McDonald. In this kind of situation, the medical instinct and training is to investigate and treat the underlying pathology, in the hope that this process will lead to some good for the patient. When this offer of help is refused, this can be hard to accept. Why is this so hard? Partly perhaps because medicine just is a very practical occupation, geared towards doing something rather than nothing. Inactivity can feel like failure. A rejection of medical attention can feel like a personal rejection of the doctor herself, given the strong identity between medical skills and personal identity. A situation like this in which the harms to the patient are so grave can severely test the limits of our commitment to patient self-determination. There is often the feeling that perhaps the patient did not understand the diagnosis, or likely consequences, or possibility for treatment. Perhaps the GP should have tried a bit harder to explain things. This is an important point: before accepting a refusal of treatment with potentially harmful consequences, we must ensure that the patient fully understands the implications of their decision.

How can we tell if a refusal is informed? The criteria for informed refusals are the same as for informed consent (see also Chapter 6 for a full discussion of informed consent).

(a) The patient must be competent to make this decision.

(b) The doctor must provide enough information so that the patient can fully understand the nature and effects of the treatment that is recommended, and the likely consequences of refusing treatment.

(c) The patient must be making the decision voluntarily, without any coercion or manipulation by other people.

Why do patients like Mrs Duke refuse treatment? There is no single answer to this question, as people will refuse different treatments for different reasons. However, in each situation where there is a risk of serious harm to the patient, it is part of good practice for the GP to ask about the patient's reasoning and try to understand why they are refusing treatment (Connelly 2000). This effort to understand on the part of the GP plays two ethical roles. First, listening to the patient demonstrates a commitment to care and trustworthiness, even though the doctor might prefer a different outcome. Secondly, by eliciting the patient's reasons for refusal, the GP can correct any misunderstandings and be satisfied that the refusal is fully informed.

If we consider the role of the patient in deciding her own good, and accept that medical care is only part of that good, refusals of treatment are a justifiable limit on beneficence. Beneficence requires that we do our best to offer medical care; patients however, are not obliged to accept our offer. Imposing care upon people who do not want it is strongly paternalistic and violates patient autonomy. Chapter 6 explores patient autonomy more fully.

Complete refusals of medical care are relatively rare. More commonly, patients partially accept medical advice.

Case 4.5

Mr Jason Allen is a 29-year-old man with moderately severe asthma. He works in a pub, and smokes 10–15 cigarettes per day. He takes regular inhaled steroids and bronchodilators, but usually requires a short course of oral steroids for exacerbations of his asthma several times per year. His GP, Dr Carter, finds it very frustrating to see Mr Allen. He cannot understand why Mr Allen will not give up smoking and find a job in a smoke-free environment.

From a medical point of view, Mr Allen's behaviour is very unsatisfactory, as he will almost certainly see an improvement in his asthma if he gives up smoking and/or changes jobs. There is a clear medical view about what is in this patient's best interests. However, Mr Allen does not follow medical advice and seems quite content to carry on smoking and to use oral steroids for his exacerbations.

What are the ethical considerations here? Dr Carter has a duty to act for the good of Mr Allen and to prevent harms, but achieving this good relies upon the patient changing his behaviour. Does Mr Allen have any obligation to follow medical advice? In general, medical ethicists have considered that patients always have the right to refuse treatment, and that there is no definite obligation to accept medical advice. This is upheld in law (Mason and McCall Smith 1999). However, part of being a trustworthy patient (as discussed in Chapter 2) is that the patient is genuinely seeking health care. In cases like that of Mr Allen, Dr Carter may find it helpful to clarify with Mr Allen what his aims are, and how these may be understood in the context of appearing to ignore medical advice. Despite the difficulty of working with patients who seem to be wilfully damaging their health, GPs are committed to providing general medical services and should not withhold services even if they feel that the patient is compromising their medical care one way or another. It might be worth asking whether Dr Carter would feel differently if Mr Allen were an enthusiastic jogger and often presented to the surgery with injuries related to his jogging? The obligation to do the best medically for the patient remains, despite any feelings of approval or disapproval about the patient's health-affecting actions.

Patients who attend frequently with illnesses that are exacerbated by their own behaviours raise questions about justice and resource allocation. If Mr Allen followed medical advice, this would decrease his need for medical services, reducing pressure on the system, and leaving Dr Carter more time to see other patients. Do citizens within a state-funded system like the NHS have an obligation to limit their demands on the available resources? It seems reasonable to say that people have a duty not to use health services carelessly or casually, as by doing this they can divert attention away from more urgent cases, for example, calling an ambulance for a sprained wrist, or calling for a home visit for a repeat prescription (Draper and Sorrell 2002). But who should be the judge of careful use? This is where the difficulties start, as fear and lack of knowledge can be potent triggers for actions that might seem unwarranted from a medical perspective. The nature of general practice offers the opportunity for GPs to discuss with patients the best way to use the health care offered by the practice. (See Chapter 5 for a full discussion of justice and resource allocation.)

ancing beneficence and autonomy

ventive care highlights the tensions that may occur between bal-
ing the two ethical duties of beneficence and respect for auto-
my. Preventive care is based upon acting for the good of the
son receiving the care, in terms of avoiding preventable harms.
is is a strong moral foundation, but can be compromised if there
undue pressures to make sure that patients comply with preven-
e care. Pressures may come from external sources, for example
vernment targets for immunizations or cervical cancer screening
at link financial rewards to rates of immunization or screening.
is creates a potential conflict of interests for the GP. To act in the
st interests of the patient requires that the GP explain the preven-
e activity and seek informed consent, with the final decision left
to the patient. However, if the patient refuses, this may affect the
P's income. Patients who realize that GPs have a financial interest
achieving preventive care targets may feel that they are coerced,
r example by receiving multiple and unsolicited reminders to
ttend for cervical cancer screening. (See also Chapter 9 on conflicts
f interest.)

Many preventive activities are routine, such as recording risk factors
r measuring blood pressure. We often take consent for granted in
hese cases, but for some preventive activities, more formal informed
onsent is critical. This can be difficult, especially when the informa-
ion is hard to assemble or equivocal, as for example the recent con-
roversies about the benefits of breast cancer screening. The concern
ver the measles–mumps–rubella vaccine highlighted the difficulties
for GPs of implementing a national immunization strategy in the face
of emotive reporting and high levels of distrust.

Preventing harms

Part of the ethical complexity of preventive care and screening lies in
trying to balance an abstract and often quite small risk for a patient
against the possible harms from the intervention. For example, lower-
ing cholesterol levels across the population will lead to a measurable
and significant decrease in heart disease, but for any one individual,
the decrease in risk may be negligible. This is the prevention paradox,

Practitioner-driven constraints and medical responsibility

Are there any limits to the extent of GPs' commitment to act for their
patients' good? We can break down the duty of beneficence into four
parts:

(a) One ought not to inflict evil or harm.

(b) One ought to prevent evil or harm.

(c) One ought to remove evil.

(d) One ought to do or promote good (Frankena 1973).

Following this account, GPs would be more obliged to prevent or
remove harms than to do good, and this ties in with our intuitions and
some empirical observations (Rogers 1999). Health care does seem to
have adopted this hierarchy with its greater obligation to act to prevent
harms than to promote good—just think of the way that medical budgets are split between acute and preventive services. But what of the limits to doing or promoting good? Does this create a potentially limitless
demand to perform supererogatory actions on behalf of patients? This
issue is particularly difficult in general practice, where there is less distinction between the patient's health interests and their overall interests
compared with secondary or tertiary care. It may be difficult to define
clear limits to medical responsibility. For almost every consultation it
is possible to think of some extra effort or action that could have bene-
fited the patient; these feelings are compounded by the time pressures operating in much of general practice.

Conflict may occur between GPs and patients if patients request medical services which GPs consider unnecessary. For example, guidelines
and reviews on the management of low back pain advise that plain
lumbar X-rays should not be performed routinely. Not only are they
unlikely to help diagnostically, there are the potential harms of inciden-
tal findings and the exposure to irradiation. From a medical perspective,
these are quite powerful reasons to refuse requests for an X-ray. But what
of the patient who, for whatever reason, is not reassured by this line of
reasoning. Perhaps they know someone who was also refused an X-ray
for back pain who turned out to have cancer, perhaps it is just not possible for that person to accept a diagnosis of soft tissue strain unless they

have seen for themselves that there is nothing wrong with their bones. GPs may often find themselves forced to choose between an externally mandated standard of care (for example a guideline) and what they feel to be in the best interests of this particular patient, based upon their personal knowledge and communication with the patient. There is no single way to resolve problems of this kind that require balancing up the various factors case by case. On the one hand there are pressures to do with practising scientific medicine, not wasting resources, and adhering to standards of care, but on the other hand, refusing a request may compromise the therapeutic relationship with the patient and fail to recognize important facts about that particular patient.

External constraints

Acting in the patient's best interests can be constrained by external circumstances, such as lack of resources to follow medically-indicated courses of actions. This is a sometimes severe problem in the NHS where patients are faced with waiting lists for investigations, referrals, and treatments. In some ways, external constraints do not cause the same ethical distress as constraints related to patients. This might be because GPs do not feel responsible for the shortcomings of the NHS in the way that they might feel responsible for some of the actions of their patients. Once a patient is waiting for some further action, pressure eases on the GP. Delays, crises, and shortcomings are accepted as part and parcel of the NHS, by patients and practitioners alike.

However, external constraints do raise ethical issues, especially when access to specialists through the NHS may take months, whilst private appointments can be obtained at very short notice. Private access to secondary and tertiary services creates a double standard of health care, with those who can afford to receiving a much swifter service. If these patients are then slotted into public operating lists, ahead of people waiting for public out-patients' appointments, the injustice is compounded.

Screening, disease prevention, and health promotion

One area of health care that raises specific questions about beneficence is preventive care. Preventive activities are now within the

mainstream business of general practice, reflec policy on prevention, which in turn refle 'Prevention is better than cure.' Why is it genera vention is better than cure? There are a number question. There are ethical reasons why preventi cure. The most important of these is that prevent of disease, and the duty of beneficence includes far as possible, harms. If we accept that health individuals are harmed by ill health, then we have try to prevent ill health. Medically speaking, then that cannot be prevented; some of these, for exa have a better prognosis the earlier that they are d also economic reasons why prevention may be b preventing disease may be cheaper than treating it nomic arguments are not infallible.

Both the ethical and the medical views about pr towards performing preventive activities, howeve ethical concerns.

Box 4.3 Ethical issues raised by preve

Balancing beneficence and autonomy

1 What pressures are there to ensure patient comp

2 Has the patient given informed consent?

Preventing harms

1 What is the balance of benefits over harms, short term?

2 How do the harms and benefits affect individuals populations?

Justice

1 Who receives the preventive care and what is the in inequalities in health?

first described by Rose: actions to improve health on the part of individuals often show a benefit at the population level but not for that particular individual (Rose 1985). When the preventive action involves making changes that are quite intrusive into the life of the patient, such as major dietary changes, we need to be certain that the benefits are worth the effort for the patient. Technical information can help to inform decisions, such as the rates of false positives and negatives, and the possible consequences of a false positive. What happens to a person with a positive test, in terms of further investigations, and how should we measure the fear and anxiety felt for example, by a person with a positive faecal occult blood test who is waiting for further investigations?

Justice: what is the impact upon inequalities in health?

One of the major ethical issues raised by preventive care and health promotion is that these activities are more likely to taken up by people living in more well-off socio-economic circumstances than by people living in more deprived circumstances (Acheson 1998). This means that although the health of some (well-off) groups may be improved, the benefits are not spread evenly and there can be a widening of the existing health gap. In addition, the focus upon the individual and their role in being healthy takes no account of the structural features of society that lead to ill health. Rather than provide an environment that supports healthy eating and exercise, the problem is medicalized and made into an issue of personal responsibility. Promoting an ethos of individual responsibility for health is unlikely to address the significant health inequalities that exist in the UK unless there are also structural changes.

Conclusion

Acting for the good of patients is one of the fundamental ethical requirements of medical practice. In this chapter we have explored some of the complexities that may arise when GPs try to act for the good of their patients, and the relationship between beneficence and paternalism. Sometimes patients themselves may act in ways that hinder their medical interests, and sometimes external circumstances can lead to less than optimal care. Health prevention activities raise their own challenges, as the expected benefits may be difficult to predict with accuracy, and following national policies on prevention may limit the informed choices of patients. Finally, we have briefly raised the issue of justice; this is explored fully in the next chapter.

References

Acheson, D. (1998). Independent inquiry into inequalities in health. The Stationery Office, London.

Christie, R. and Hoffmaster, B. (1986). *Ethical issues in family medicine.* Oxford University Press, New York, NY.

Connelly, J. (2000). Refusal of treatment. In Sugarman, J. (ed.) *Ethics in primary care.* McGraw-Hill, New York, NY.

Downie, R. and Calman, K. (1994). *Healthy respect: ethics in health care,* (2nd edn). Oxford University Press, Oxford.

Draper, H. and Sorrell, T. (2002). Patients' responsibilities in medical ethics. *Bioethics* 16, 335–52.

General Medical Council (2001). *Duties of a doctor. http://www.gmc-uk.org/ standards/standards_frameset.htm*

Jacobson, L., Edwards, A., Granier, S., and Butler, C. (1997). Evidence-based medicine and general practice. *British Journal of General Practice* 47, 449–52.

Katz, J. (1984). *The silent world of doctor and patient.* Free Press, New York, NY.

Mason, J. and McCall Smith, R. (1999). *Law and medical ethics,* (5th edn). Butterworths, London.

Rogers, W. A. (1999). Beneficence in general practice: an empirical investigation. *Journal of Medical Ethics* 25 (5), 388–93.

Rogers, W. A. (2002). Are guidelines ethical? Some considerations for general practice. *British Journal of General Practice* 52, 663–9.

Rose, G. (1985). Sick individuals and sick populations. *International Journal of Epidemiology* 14, 32–8.

Savage, R. and Armstrong, D. (1990). Effect of a general practitioner's consulting style on patients' satisfaction: a controlled study. *British Medical Journal* 301, 968–70.

Sherwin, S. (1992). *No longer patient: feminist ethics and health care.* Temple University Press, Philadelphia, PA.

Thomas, K. (1987). General practice consultations: is there any point in being positive? *British Medical Journal* 294, 1200–2.

Watt, G. (2002). The inverse care law today. *Lancet* 360, 252–4.

Further reading

Connelly, J. (2000). Refusal of treatment. In Sugerman, J. (ed.) *Ethics in primary care.* McGraw-Hill, New York, NY.

Health Care Analysis (2002). **10** (3). Special issue: *Into the hidden world behind evidence-based medicine.* This is a series of articles analysing some of the ethical issues raised by evidence-based medicine.

Pellegrino, E. D. and Thomasma, D. (1988). *For the patient's good: the restoration of beneficence in health care.* Oxford University Press, New York, NY.

Rogers, W. A. (1999). Beneficience in general practice: an empirical investigation. *Journal of Medical Ethics* **25** (5), 388–93.

Rogers, W. A. (2002). Are guidelines ethical? Some considerations for general practice. *British Journal of Medical Practice* **52**, 663–9.

Sherwin, S. (1992). *No longer patient.* Temple University Press, Philadelphia, PA.

Chapter 5

Justice and resource allocation in general practice

Case 5.1

Dr Martin Schroeder occasionally works in the Hackney Road Practice in inner city London. Jennifer is Dr Schroeder's sixth appointment this morning. He has only met Jennifer once before, but he can tell immediately that Jennifer seems tired and flat. Yet, Jennifer's reasons for presenting seem very minor. She's worried that a fall three months ago on the steps outside her house may be the reason she can not conceive. She already has two children, each conceived after a year of trying. She and her partner have been trying to get pregnant for six months now. After examining her, and finding no evidence of any effects of the fall, Dr Schroeder tries to reassure Jennifer that a minor fall is unlikely to stop her conceiving. He suggests that Jennifer return at the end of the year if she is still not pregnant and her regular doctor can begin some investigations then. On the tip of Dr Schroeder's tongue are the words: "You seem very down in the dumps, Jennifer.

Case 5.1 *(Cont.)*

Is anything else troubling you?" but, Dr Schroeder is already running 30 minutes late, and he has a busy clinic still ahead of him. He tells himself: "Maybe I'm not being fair to her, but if I get further behind now, I'll never catch up. And, she'll come back again if there's really something wrong."

Case 5.2

Dr Carter scans the day's appointments. He notices Mr Servante has another appointment for 10.00 and his heart sinks. Mr Servante's multiple problems (headaches, irritable bowel syndrome, joint pains, tiredness) always have to be dealt with immediately. He is usually worried that Dr Carter is hiding something from him and so he refuses to leave until Dr Carter has slowly and carefully explained every detail. Dr Carter expects to be running at least one hour late by the time Mr Servante leaves. "It's not fair", he thinks to himself. "Every other patient I see today suffers because of him."

Case 5.3

Dr Day has known Simone since she was 10, when he first joined the practice. Now Simone is 25, a secretary in the local solicitor's office. She is an attractive woman but, from her point of view, she has one major problem: her nose. Simone's nose is large and she believes it completely disfigures her face. She is convinced that the reason she can not attract and keep a boyfriend is because no man will look twice at someone with a nose her size.

Since Simone first raised this issue with him about five years ago Dr Day has come to understand that, for whatever reason, Simone's nose really does impact significantly on her life. She is often depressed and she presents regularly with ill-defined aches and pains that never really seem to resolve. He has facilitated access to counselling, but this has not really helped. In fact, the psychologist implied that cosmetic surgery might indeed be a good solution for Simone's problems. At her urging, Dr Day has tried to get Simone in to see a plastic surgeon to have her assessed. But here's the problem: the local health authority does not fund cosmetic surgery except for a small number of very limited conditions, so Simone will not be able to have cosmetic surgery within the NHS.

Today Simone is sitting in front of Dr Day in tears. He has just told her that, if she wants her nose fixed, she will need to be treated in the private sector. Both of them know this is unrealistic, for Simone's means are modest. "It's just not fair", she sobs, "Isn't there anything we can do about it?"

This chapter is about allocating resources fairly in a general practice setting. Our examples set the scene. Although they are very different, in each case people are concerned that 'it's not fair'. But, when we talk about things as being fair or unfair, just or unjust, what do we mean? And how can we decide what the 'fair' or 'just' thing might be?

Problems such as these can pose troubling dilemmas for many doctors (GMC 1999). Resolution of resource allocation dilemmas can be assisted by a thoughtful consideration of the ways in which decisions are being made, and an analysis of the criteria for a just distribution. This chapter deals with these issues. We begin with a definition of resource allocation and an account of the many ways in which resources are currently shared out in the NHS. This is followed by a philosophical discussion of theories and principles of justice, focusing on four criteria for the allocation of health care resources—allocation according to need, capacity to benefit, merit, and rights.

What is resource allocation and why does it matter?

Resource allocation involves the distribution of goods and services to people, programmes, or projects. In health care, resource allocation takes place at a number of levels. At the level of *macroallocation*, it concerns decisions, often made by government or health officials, about which programmes will be supported and to what degree. Such decisions are not limited to health care; they also concern how much to allocate to other social goods, such as housing, education, and transport. Programmes outside the 'health budget' will often have impacts on health; for example, transport policy can impact on health through decisions about road upgrades and the presence of speed cameras.

Within the health budget, decisions need to be made about how to allocate the available monies. So, for example, governments must make decisions about the degree of emphasis they place on health promotion and preventive services for children, as opposed to, say, care and treatment services for children who have life-threatening illnesses.

At the level of *mesoallocation,* resource allocation decisions are made within institutions. How will the local hospital distribute its budget between the various services it provides? Should the local health authority support an intensive visiting programme for new mothers and their babies? On a smaller scale, general practitioners also make mesoallocation decisions, for example, when the topic of the practice meeting turns to the distribution of the practice budget. Do we employ a second health visitor, or would it be better to have a full-time accountant? Simone is a 'victim' of mesoallocation rationing decisions; her local health authority has decided that, with a limited budget available, it will not commission the cosmetic surgery services that would benefit Simone.

Microallocation decisions relate to individual patients. In general practice, problems of microallocation occur, for instance, when a GP has to decide if she will make an important house call first, or see that patient who has been in the waiting room for the last hour. Both Dr Schroeder and Dr Carter are making microallocation decisions when they decide either to cut short a potentially lengthy consultation or to allow a consultation to run on.

What all these situations have in common is that there is not enough money, time, staff, machines, or other resources available to do everything for every patient. Butler puts the problem in this way:

> Whether care is organized as a tax-funded service that is free at the point of use or as a commercial enterprise for which people pay directly or through insurance, it is simply not possible to offer the full spectrum of clinical possibilities to every patient at every stage of life. The cost would be unsustainable, whether it fell on citizens as tax-payers or on patients as fee-payers.
>
> (Butler 1999, p. 6)

Scarcity is thus an inevitable characteristic of any health system.

Although a GP's prime responsibility is to the individual patient (RCGP 2002), there are at least two reasons why GPs can not avoid resource allocation issues completely. First, scarcity is a characteristic of many of the services GPs themselves provide. As we have seen above, it is often the GPs' *time* that is the scarce resource. In addition, general practitioners have a crucial role to play in resource allocation decisions beyond their own practices because they are often 'gatekeepers' to other services offered within the health care system. GPs stand at the gate to health services, deciding who should be let through. In addition, they use their professional judgement to decide which treatments and services are warranted for which patients.

When GPs use both their own resources and those they gatekeep wastefully, less resources are available for their patients and for those of other doctors (RCGP 2002, p. 12).

How are resources allocated in the NHS?

Before we turn to a discussion of principles and theories of justice, it is worth noting the range of rationing options that are used on a daily basis. Butler (1999) provides a list of the strategies that are actually used within the NHS. First, he suggests that one way governments can address the problem of rationing health services and treatment is by being explicit about their health care priorities. This approach has been used in Britain for a long time, for example, from the NHS's stated priority for the elderly and the mentally ill in the 1970s, through to setting targets for morbidity and mortality in specific disease areas in the 1990s. Whether this priority setting approach has worked is

Box 5.1 The range of rationing approaches used in the NHS

Influences on supply

1 Articulating explicit priorities for health care.

2 Removing services from the menu of those on offer.

3 Relying on the courts.

Influences on demand

1 Reducing the demand for care by discouraging people from entering the system.

2 Reducing the demand for care by slowing people's progress through the system.

3 Enhancing the efficiency and effectiveness of care.

4 Refocusing attention towards prevention.

5 Devolving rationing responsibility to clinicians.

(Adapted from Butler 1999, pp. 16–36.)

another matter; there is some evidence to suggest that, despite encouragement from central government to address priorities explicitly, local health authorities have not shifted resources from areas of lower priority to areas of higher priority.

A second way in which the rationing problem is addressed within the NHS is to remove some services completely, and to shift the resources that would be allocated to these services to others. For example, local health authorities do make decisions to drop certain treatments off the list of services that they make available to patients in their regions; the most common ones have been 'reversal of female sterilization, in vitro fertilization, sex change operations, breast augmentation, rhinoplasty, the reversal of male vasectomy, the removal of tattoos, and cosmetic surgery for varicose veins' (Butler 1999, p. 21). When health authorities in the UK exclude treatments from their list of services, they appear to make decisions either because there is relevant scientific evidence available (for example, excluding ear grommets) or because it seems that the desired treatment or service is a matter of private preference rather than health need (for example, cosmetic surgery). Regardless of the reasons, very little debate about these issues seems to take place in the public sphere.

A third way in which rationing decisions occur is to try to rely on the courts. However, despite a number of test cases in recent years, the courts have tended to avoid making legal judgements in this arena, preferring to regard such decisions as the proper responsibility of government, health authorities, and clinicians.

The strategies considered so far have focused on the supply side of the rationing problem. The other alternative open to those who need to ration health services is to alter the demand for services. Butler suggests that we can influence demand for health care in two ways: we can try to discourage patients from entering the health care system (primary inhibitors), and we can slow down patients' progress once they are in the system (secondary inhibitors).

In the NHS, primary inhibitors work principally through GPs, since, as noted above, GPs are the gateway to most health care. Examples of primary inhibitors are education campaigns for patients on sensible use of your GP, reception practices (answering services, triaging by reception staff, etc.), and appointment systems (which create a delay between a patient's intention to seek treatment and the service itself so that some people drop out in this period).

Once in the system, secondary inhibitors function to control demand. Delay in access to out-patient appointments, or admission as in-patients, is a well-known phenomenon to any GP. Denial involves doctors and others simply refusing to acknowledge that the delayed or unavailable service would actually be of benefit to the patient. Dilution makes the services available but spreads it so thinly that each person get a less than desirable service (Parker 1975). For example, fertility treatment may be restricted to one or two cycles. Another strategy in this stable is to dilute the expertise of staff, by employing more junior staff, or differently and less qualified staff to deliver the service.

The sixth strategy used in the NHS to ration services is to try to enhance the efficiency and effectiveness of the system. 'Efficiency . . . is about maximizing the quantity and quality of what is achieved from a given quantum of resource' (Butler 1999, p. 31). Effectiveness, on the other hand, is not related to cost, but rather to how well a treatment works, usually when compared against other treatments. The rise of evidence-based medicine (discussed in Chapter 4) is a direct result of efforts to attend to both the efficiency and effectiveness of particular treatments. Evidence-based medicine will not, however, necessarily reduce the health care budget. For example, if we find a treatment to be effective, the pressure for it to be available to all will be considerable, regardless of the availability of resources to fund it.

A seventh way to manage the rationing problem is to refocus health care so that problems are prevented before they arise. We have discussed this issue in Chapter 4. Ethically, the arguments are complex, as prevention can often mean more paternalism on the part of government or doctors.

The final strategy that Butler notes is to devolve allocation decisions to clinicians. On a daily basis, GPs make many decisions about the allocation of resources.

> It is as though there exists an unspoken social contract: 'society' has entrusted to the clinicians the responsibility for taking the ultimate decisions about the allocation of scarce resources, and in return 'society' has absolved the clinicians from explicit democratic accountability for their stewardship of that responsibility.

(Butler 1999, p. 35)

Mostly, such decisions happen with little awareness amongst the public more generally, although occasionally the popular press brings the attention of the general community to specific decisions.

Listing the range of ways that rationing currently takes place within the NHS is one thing; deciding whether such approaches are fair and morally acceptable is a different task altogether. Clearly, not all of these approaches to resource allocation are of equal moral worth and the breadth and variety of strategies only reinforces the need for a rational and sound basis for distributing scarce health care resources. The rest of this chapter draws on principles and theories of justice to help us analyse different ways to allocate resources.

How can we allocate resources fairly?

Theories and principles of justice

At its most simple, justice is done when each person gets his or her due. This suggests that people who are equal with respect to their 'dues' ought to get the same amount. Indeed, all theories of justice, from Aristotle onwards, have had as a minimum formal requirement that equals shall be treated equally and unequals unequally. This is a 'formal' principle of justice, because it provides no detail about the circumstances under which equals should be treated equally and because it does not tell us whether two or more people are in fact equal.

Fleshing out the formal principle of justice is the chief issue in debates about distributive justice. Just what criteria can we use to decide whether people are equal or unequal? What is it about Mr Servante that makes Dr Carter think it unfair that he take up more surgery time than other patients? Should Simone be regarded as equal to other patients who have different treatment needs or wishes?

Box 5.2 Formal principle of justice

The formal principle of justice states that equals shall be treated equally and unequals unequally.

We need a way to flesh out or give content to this formal principle of justice. There are really two routes we can take. The first route focuses on processes or procedures that we may use to allocate resources—this leads us to considerations of *procedural justice*. The second route concerns the characteristics of individuals or groups to whom resources may go and the outcomes resulting from that distribution. This route leads to the identification of *material principles of justice*.

Procedural justice

Procedural justice approaches the problem of fairness by suggesting that we can arrive at fair or just outcomes if the procedures that we use to allocate our resources are fair. One famous example of procedural justice is John Rawls' 'veil of ignorance' (Rawls 1972). Rawls asks us to imagine that we are in the hypothetical situation of deciding how to allocate a range of primary social goods (such as education and health care) in a society. He gives us total knowledge of the society that we are making decisions for, *but* we have absolutely no knowledge of what our personal position will be in that society. Behind this 'veil of ignorance', Rawls suggests that reasonable decision-makers will be able to allocate resources in a fair way.

Generally, fair procedures in health care will not guarantee fair outcomes, but they will help. At a broad societal level, for example, citizens' referenda and community consultations have been used occasionally to decide which services will be provided within a geographical region. At more local levels, fair procedures can contribute significantly to fair outcomes. For example, the ways in which research ethics committees make decisions about which research will be allowed to proceed and which will not are significantly enhanced when the committee's activities are demonstrably impartial, transparent to interested parties, and clear.

Material principles of justice

Philosophers label the ways that we give content to our formal principle of justice *material principles* of justice. These principles provide criteria that we can use to determine who should be entitled to receive the resources that are available. In a sense, they give us a range of standards that we may use to measure equality (or inequality) amongst people.

Different scholars offer different alternatives for material principles of justice. In this chapter, we will consider:

(a) Allocation of health resources according to need.

(b) Allocation of health resources according to capacity to benefit.

(c) Allocation of health resources according to merit.

(d) Allocation of health resources according to rights.

Obviously, the corollary of these statements is that people who have different needs, or capacity to benefit, or merit, or rights should be treated differently.

Box 5.3 Material principles of justice

1 Health care resources should be allocated according to need.

2 Health care resources should be allocated according to capacity to benefit.

3 Health care resources should be allocated according to merit.

4 Health care resources should be allocated according to rights.

In the following section we examine each of these alternatives and explore their strengths and weaknesses.

Choosing between people on the basis of need

The first way in which we can choose between people when allocating health resources is to allocate according to need. It seems obvious that people with equal need should have equal access to resources and, indeed, treatment on the basis of clinical need has been at the core of the NHS since its inception. Allocating according to clinical need such that people who are sick get treated and the sickest get treated first has always been a guiding principle for doctors.

Yet, beneath this apparent simplicity lies a myriad of problems. 'Need' as a concept is hard to grasp firmly, in part because 'need' and 'want' are not always distinct. There are circumstances in which the two are clearly differentiated—for example, a patient's need for surgery to treat acute appendicitis is of a rather different order to his desire to be in a private room during his hospital stay. But there are other circumstances in which need and want are not so easy to distinguish. Cosmetic surgery such as that desired by Simone raises particularly sharply the confusion between needs and wants. When does a disfiguring nose become so significant that the desire to have a smaller nose become a legitimate health need? Dr Carter may also be thinking about the relationship between needs and desires when he grumbles about Mr Servante's lengthy consultations. From Dr Carter's point of view, Mr Servante may have a great desire for reassurance, but his actual need for treatment is fairly minor and probably less than other patients in the waiting room. If Dr Carter could organize his clinic so that he is treating according to need, Mr Servante would receive less time and other patients more.

The example of Dr Carter and Mr Servante raises a second problem for needs-based resource allocation. Just who should decide which needs are legitimate? This issue can be addressed to some extent by distinguishing between subjective and objective needs. Subjective needs are the needs that people define themselves as having. Objective needs are defined by someone else, often specific categories of people who have the authority to make judgements about the severity of need. In our society, doctors are authorized to make decisions about whether a patient's need is objectively real or not.

We might think that using a subjective needs-based criterion for the allocation of health resources would always result in patients wanting more than the GP might think reasonable and, conversely, that if we leave the judgement of need up to GPs, they will always deliver less than patients want. Certainly, this is what would seem to be happening in Mr Servante's case. However, Dr Schroeder's interaction with Jennifer casts this issue in a different light. Here it is Dr Schroeder who is second-guessing an unacknowledged need in Jennifer. Dr Schroeder is using a rationing schema here that, at least partly, allocates GP time according to need only when the patient explicitly acknowledges her need. In daily practice, much of the resource allocating that GPs do is probably of this nature; it is a see-saw between patient-led identification of need and GP-led response to acknowledged need.

Even if doctor and patient can agree on the severity of the need, there are other problems for needs-based resource allocation. What are we to make of the fact that a significant proportion of the conditions GPs see just improve of their own accord over time? We might argue that these conditions could hardly be said to 'need' treatment at all. In these circumstances, should patients with these conditions be seen in GP surgeries at all? Or, would it be fairer to those patients with 'real' needs if minor self-limiting illnesses were assessed in other settings?

The final problem for needs-based allocation schemas is one that is noted by Butler (1999 pp. 128–33). 'Needs' may not be easily recognized outside of the resources that are available to meet them. Butler describes the case of an elderly woman with poor bladder control who is unable, because of arthritis, to get to the toilet quickly. She needs incontinence pads, but there is a local health authority policy that provides pads free of charge only to people with 'very debilitating illnesses' or as a complication of surgery. As this woman falls into neither of these categories, and because she is poor, she is often wet and has skin sores. In this situation, her need is for district nursing care for her skin sores. However, she would be better served if her need for incontinence pads, or for the money to buy them, could be met.

Sometime needs for health care arise out of situations that really demand other sorts of responses. For example, depression in a young, unemployed male might be better dealt with by finding him a job than by anti-depressants. If the 'real' need can not be met by the NHS, should the NHS meet the 'substitute' need at all? Some of the underlying causes of ill health do not lie in domains for which the NHS has responsibility (for example, poor housing). Here the NHS is reduced to dealing with the consequences rather than the causes of ill health. How do we decide which services are legitimately the responsibility of the NHS and which services fall outside its reach?

All of this suggests that need is not an all or nothing phenomenon—it is, as Butler suggests, an 'elastic' notion, that expands and contracts according to the social and economic environment. So, to allocate health services according to need is not at all straightforward.

So far in talking about health needs we have focused on deciding between individuals. When we shift our attention away from choices between individuals and to the way in which we organize the health system, we can no longer rely on doctors and patients together arriving at some sort of tacit agreement about how needs are to be judged. Allocating health resources across a system requires a more explicit approach to the identification of need. Len Doyal (1995) has attempted to do this. The value of his work for our discussion here is that he relates his theory explicitly to the organization and delivery of care within the NHS.

Doyal starts from the presumption that we can legitimately describe health care as a need, because good health is central to human flourishing. Not only do we need good health to do what we want to do with our lives for ourselves, we also need good health to be good citizens and help others fulfil their goals for themselves.

Box 5.4 Criteria for the allocation of health care resources according to need

1 Ration care within, rather than across, different categories of treatment.
2 Rank individuals according to the impact their illness or disability has on their capacity for human flourishing.
3 Randomize as a last resort.

Pre-conditions

4 Do not spend scarce resources on ineffective treatments.
5 Lifestyle should not be relevant to our chances of getting the treatment we need.
6 Debate allocation issues openly and rationally.
7 There should be mechanisms to take account of the views of the community.

(Adapted from Doyal 1995.)

Just what would a fair way to allocate the health care resources we need look like, according to Doyal? Doyal has seven principles. First, we should ration care within, rather than across, different categories of treatment. To do this, first we need to work out the cost of the total demand for health care for a particular period of time. If the available funding is, say, 70% of this total, the fairest way to allocate is to cut health care services by 30% across the board. This criterion has been criticized because, in practice, it is difficult to allocate services neatly into one category or another. Is a weight loss clinic for example, an obesity service or a cardiovascular disease service? Doyal's criterion is also unavoidably backward-looking as it is based on existing treatments and services. What if a new service becomes available? How do we incorporate it into our system?

Nonetheless, having made a certain amount of resources available within each category of care, we still have to decide between possible recipients. Doyal argues that we should rank individuals according to the impact that their illness or disability has on their capacity to flourish as human beings. Highest priority then goes to life-threatening illness, with lowest priority to treatments that we might like, but which do not really change our capacity to flourish (e.g. some forms of cosmetic surgery). Many general practices do in fact have a system for allocating access to consultations that is something like this. A practice may have a one hour block each morning to which patients who perceive an urgent need for medical treatment may come. For other, less urgent, conditions, there may be a waiting period of a few days before an appointment can be secured.

Once we have ranked people according to need, we may still be left having to choose between individuals. At this point, Doyal would advocate random allocation. Waiting lists are a form of random allocation, since there is some unpredictability about the moment that health problems strike us and prompt us to seek treatment.

Doyal's last four principles are really 'pre-conditions' (Butler 1999). We should not spend scarce resources on unproven treatments; lifestyle should not influence our chances of getting the treatment we need; we should debate allocation issues openly and rationally; and there should be mechanisms to take account of the views of the community.

Choosing between people on the basis of capacity to benefit

A second way to choose between people when allocating health resources is to focus on patients' capacity to benefit from a treatment. One of the reasons we decide not to pay for some interventions in some people is because it is considered unlikely that the person will receive any benefit from it. Sometimes this is an easy conclusion to reach, for example a person with disseminated cancer and severe cardiovascular disease is very unlikely to benefit from a coronary artery bypass graft. However, most decisions are not clear-cut—patterns of health and illness are notoriously difficult to predict at an individual level and it can be impossible to say that a person will not get *any* benefit from a particular intervention. The increasing use of EBM has led to more information about the statistical effectiveness of interventions, and this is increasingly used to control access to some services, but the question about the effectiveness in individuals remains. Mason and McCall Smith draw attention to the language that doctors use in rationing decisions with the phrase 'not clinically indicated' (1999, p. 304). This can mean either that the intervention is not likely to benefit the patient, or that the use of the intervention in this patient is not considered a worthwhile use of resources. This kind of ambivalence can provide an indirect or perhaps easier way of refusing services, but may conceal the real reasons behind the refusal.

Evidence about the effectiveness of particular interventions has become increasingly influential through the activities of NICE, which operates with the dual aims of reducing expenditure on ineffective interventions, and ensuring equal access to effective interventions. There has been much debate about the political nature of decisions made by NICE, but the attempt to provide transparency in decisions about resource allocation is to be welcomed.

Considerable attention in health economics has been paid to the issue of trying to measure capacity to benefit. The Quality Adjusted Life Year (QALY) is a measure which attempts to combine both the quantity and quality of life gained from a treatment in a single measure. The basic idea of a QALY is straightforward: one year of perfect health life expectancy is valued at 1, one year of less than perfect health life expectancy is valued at less than 1, and death is zero. A treatment which gives six months extra life at perfect health would be scored at 0.5, whereas a treatment giving one year of extra life in health which is only 25% of optimal health would be scored at 0.25. QALYs can provide an indication of the benefits gained from a variety of different medical procedures in terms of both quality of life and survival for the patient. The costs of different treatments can then be compared by looking at the costs per QALYs.

In theory, the use of QALYs can help in comparisons between competing treatments. For example if a Trust has £2 million to spend on new interventions, what kind of QALY gains can be expected from putting the money into hip replacements versus spending on asthma or coronary artery grafting? There has been much discussion about the uses and abuses of QALYs, and here we comment on two aspects. The first is apparent difficulties with economic information. If we look at just one example, that of estimating the cost-effectiveness of beta interferons and glatiramer acetate in the treatment of multiple sclerosis, the information is very confusing. Initial estimates of costs per QALY between £38 000–£106 000 almost double with methodological changes in the analysis, such as changes in the discount rates for costs and benefits (ScHARR 2001). These large variations indicate the lack of precision in economic estimates and the importance of methodological assumptions. Given the difficulties in ascribing accurate costs per QALY, it is concerning when decisions about resource allocation rely very heavily upon what can only ever be fairly imprecise estimates.

Perhaps the more concerning problem with QALYs is the attempt to quantify the value of life in terms of degree of health. The assumption is that life in poor health is less worth living than life in perfect health. This assumption immediately discriminates against people with any kind of disability or chronic health problem, as they cannot gain the same QALY benefit from an intervention as a person without disability or chronic illness. Each person's life is valuable to him or herself, even if they are not in perfect health. The question posed by QALYs seems unanswerable except at a personal level, and even at this level it is hard to imagine how a choice could be made: how would you value one year of life at 50% health (whatever that means) compared with six months at full health?

Choosing between people on the basis of merit or desert

A third way to choose between people when health services are scarce is to focus on merit or desert as a criterion. When we speak of people deserving or meriting things, we imply that their contribution, effort, or status is important and ought to be taken into account when resources are allocated. On the face of it, this seems a reprehensible way to allocate health services. Surely we ought not to give people preferential treatment just because they are wealthy, or a member of parliament, or a promising young gymnast! However, as we shall see, the merit criterion often plays a role when health services are rationed and, sometimes, it is hard to argue against its place.

Box 5.5 Examples of merit-based criteria for the allocation of health care resources

Criteria related to character

1 Grateful patients.

2 Compliant patients.

Criteria related to social role

3 Past role (e.g. World War II veteran).

4 Present role (e.g. single mother with dependent children).

5 Future role (e.g. a young person).

There are a number of ways we can conceive of merit or desert operating as a criterion for allocating health care. First, we can imagine allocating health care to people according to their personal appeal or characteristics. Should personality traits be relevant to the allocation of health care resources? There is always the temptation in general practice to focus attention on patients who are appropriately grateful for what we do for them. Personal appeal ought to be morally unacceptable, but it sometimes turns out to be the reason we treat people differently. Ethical stewarding of resources in general practice attempts to guard against such behaviour.

It is easy to show that allocating resources in general practice on the basis of how 'nice' people are is not acceptable and should not occur. However, it gets a bit harder when the character traits become 'being cooperative' or 'trying hard'. Patients' interest in and capacity to comply with treatment does have a practical influence on how much call they have on scarce health care services. For example, should a GP encourage a 42-year-old overweight smoker with asthma to join the practice Stop Smoking Clinic, even when he knows that all advice just goes in one ear and out the other? According to a needs-based argument, this patient needs the GP's time and support far more than other, more compliant, patients do. A character-based allocation of resources may be behind Dr Schroeder's consultation with Jennifer. Jennifer may just happen to be a reserved, quiet person who does not offer much information but, if invited, is willing to talk. Should reticent patients be discriminated against because they find it harder to raise problems with their GP? To what extent does Dr Schroeder have an obligation to make it as easy for Jennifer to discuss her problems as it is for a more garrulous, extroverted patient?

The problem with this version of merit-based resource allocation is that it is rather difficult to put together an argument for treating people differently based purely on their character. As Butler suggests, the case for treating nice (or responsive or extroverted) people preferentially rests upon the assumption that they have, in some sense, done something that ought to be rewarded or, at least, not punished (Butler 1999, p. 52). The idea of allocating resources according to desert makes sense only when people can do something to influence their desert, rather like training hard to win the prize at the end of a race. But, people are often unable to influence those characteristics that seem to make them deserving or undeserving of health care. The real problem with this version of the merit criterion is that the link between character, actions, and free will is actually very complex. Continuing smoking, for example, is more than a personal choice. It is also a result of clever advertising, peer pressure, and the extremely addictive qualities of nicotine. In addition, smoking-related illness often strikes in life at a point far removed from the decision to take up smoking. How much responsibility should people have to bear for decisions they may have made decades earlier?

There is a second way in which merit-based criteria for the allocation of health resources can be interpreted. This involves considering the social roles that people play and taking these roles into account when resources are allocated. Here, we can take into account people's current role, their past contribution, or their potential for contribution in the future.

We can think of examples that would fit each category. For example, if we are thinking about people's current role, we might argue that, all other things being equal, a mother with three dependent children should take priority over a 35-year-old bachelor, when it comes to access to health services. If we take into account people's past contribution, this would allow us to discriminate in favour of people who have in the past contributed significantly to society, perhaps through their service to the community, or their work as a distinguished scientist. Finally, if we look ahead to the future, we may discriminate against the elderly in favour of the young, on the basis that the young are likely to benefit society in years to come whereas the elderly have little to offer.

Such judgements are sometimes pounced on by the media. There have been a number of celebrated cases in the UK where decisions about access to scarce, often expensive, treatment appear to have been made on the basis of social roles. While this may seem to be a long way from general practice, there are many situations in which social role does influence resource allocation in general practice settings. For example, some surgeries limit the time that parents with young children wait before they see the GP, implying that there is something about being a child that is relevant to your access to the GP. Or, patients who can afford to pay may be encouraged to seek physiotherapy in the private sector, whereas poorer patients are not necessarily told that this is an option.

Introducing these alternatives reframes the question of the merit criterion as one of the place of social contribution in decision-making about resource allocation. Again, in this arena, the tricky issues of free will and responsibility rear their heads. Just how able are we to make ourselves socially valuable people? Issues such as these are inevitably controversial, and explicit discussion of them is often swept under the carpet. The point we wish to make here is that merit criteria for resource allocation are often used unconsciously or appear disguised as other reasons. Such a situation is undesirable. If we are to use such social worth criteria, the debate about their applicability needs to occur in the open and in a constructive manner.

Choosing between people on the basis of rights

There is a lot of talk about a 'right to health care', much of it rather confusing. What does it mean to say that people have a right to health care? Does having a right to health care include having a right to cosmetic surgery because you think, as Simone does, that your nose is unattractive? Or is having a right to health care having only a right to emergency surgery? What about Mr Servante's right to have his questions answered fully?

In the United Kingdom, debate about the right to health care has usually played second fiddle to discussion of clinical need. This is because the NHS has been based on the core principle that it 'will provide a universal service for all based on clinical need, not ability to pay' (National Health Service 2000). This is not necessarily the case in other countries, notably in the United States of America, in which debate about resource allocation tends to focus mainly on rights. Still, it is important to introduce the concept of a right to health care here, if only in brief.

Some rights are described as basic human rights. For example, there are rights to be allowed to do things, to be free of interference (rights to life, liberty, and property). There are also rights to be given things (for example, rights to employment and subsistence, food, clothing, housing, or medical care). These rights are the content of statements such as the Universal Declaration of Human Rights.

There is a second kind of right that is linked more closely to the way the society we live in is organized. Some rights are acquired through agreements, contracts, or promises that we are party to. These contracts or promises can take a variety of forms, from those which have the full force of the law behind them (for example, my right as a pedestrian to expect cars to stop for me at pedestrian crossings is protected by traffic laws) to those that are merely established forms of behaviour, where no explicit promises have been made (for example, the right of a child to care and concern by her parents). When patients register with a general practice, they have a right to receive primary care from that practice, and behind this right sits the agreements that the staff of the practice have made with government.

In the United Kingdom, there is, to some degree, a right to health care in both of the senses identified above. We can describe the right to health care as a basic right. The difficulty with thinking about a right in this way is that it does not make clear just who is obligated to attend to the right to health care. The person or persons with the obligation to provide care remain shadowy characters, sometimes taking the form of 'the NHS' or 'the health authority'.

To be clear about who is obliged to provide the service, we need to turn to our second definition of a right. If we focus on a right to health care as a contract or promise, then it is easier to identify the individuals and groups who have a duty to provide health care. For GPs, this issue is most relevant in the context of their relationship with the patients registered with their practice. Many practices have a statement of patient rights, which will include such things as:

(a) Confidentiality from all members of staff.

(b) Courteous treatment by all staff.

(c) Access to personal medical records.

(d) An appointment the same day for acute illnesses.

(e) An appointment within a week for non-acute illnesses.

(f) Complaints mechanisms that are enforced.

With respect to these rights, the obligation to meet patient expectations lies with the GPs and other practice staff. Implicit in these statements is the assumption that all patients registered with the practice have the same right of access to services.

Conclusion

In this chapter we have explored a range of issues that arise because of the problem of scarcity in health care. We have reviewed the range of ways in which resource allocation decisions are made in the NHS, and considered the four main contenders for a just allocation of health resources—allocation according to need, to capacity to benefit, to merit, and to rights. Our discussion of these issues grew out of the consideration of the principle of beneficence in Chapter 4. In the next chapter we return to issues more directly concerned with the care of individual patients, with a discussion of patient autonomy in general practice.

References

Butler, J. (1999). *The ethics of health care rationing: principles and practices.* Cassell, London.

Doyal, L. (1995). Needs, rights and equity: moral quality in healthcare rationing. *Quality in Health Care* **4**, 273–83.

General Medical Council (1999). *Management in health care: the role of doctors.* General Medical Council, London. *http://www.gmc-uk.org/standards/default.htm*

Mason, J. and McCall Smith, R. (1999). *Law and medical ethics* (5th edn). Butterworths, London.

National Health Service. *Your guide to the NHS.* Accessed at *http://www.nhs.uk/nhsguide/home.htm*, March 19, 2003.

Parker, R.A. (1975). Social administration and scarcity. In Butterworth, E. and Holman, R. (ed.) *Social welfare in modern Britain,* pp. 204–12. Fontana Collins, Glasgow.

Rawls, J. (1972). *A theory of justice.* Oxford University Press, Oxford.

Royal College of General Practitioners/General Practitioners Committee (British Medical Association) (2002). *Good medical practice for general practitioners.* RCGP, London.

ScHARR. (2001). Cost effectiveness of beta interferons and glatiramer acetate in the management of multiple sclerosis. Final report to the National Institute for Clinical Excellence. ScHARR, Sheffield. *http://www.nice.org.uk/pdf/msscharreport.pdf*

Further Reading

Beauchamp, T.L. and Faden, R.R. (1979). The right to health and the right to health care. *Journal of Medicine and Philosophy* **4**, 118–131.

Butler, J. (1999). *The ethics of health care rationing. Principles and practices.* Cassell, London.

Daniels, N. (1985). *Just health care.* Cambridge University Press, New York, NY.

Doyal, L. (1995). Needs, rights and equity: moral quality in healthcare rationing. *Quality in Health Care* **4**, 273–83.

Feinberg, J. (1973). *Social philosophy.* Prentice-Hall Inc, Englewood Cliffs, NJ.

Frost, B.R. (1997). Gatekeepers no more: family practitioners as power brokers and fence wanderers. *New Zealand Medical Journal* **110**, 129–130.

General Medical Council (1999). *Management in healthcare: the role of doctors.* General Medical Council, London. *http://www.gmc-uk.org/standards/default.htm.*

Miller, D. (1979). *Social justice.* Clarendon Press, Oxford.

Rawls, J. (1972). *A theory of justice.* Oxford University Press, Oxford.

Chapter 6

Making decisions: patient autonomy in general practice

Introduction

Case 6.1

Grace Hopkins is a 54-year-old woman with mild to moderate osteoarthritis of both knees, for which she takes regular non-steroidal anti-inflammatories. Grace also has a past history of a meniscal tear followed by arthroscopy for partial removal of cartilage in her right knee. She comes to see her GP, Dr Imogen Jones, for medical advice prior to going trekking for three weeks in Nepal. Grace wishes to know what the likely effect of the trekking will be, and if there is anything that she can do to

Case 6.1 *(Cont.)*

minimize the damage to her knees. Dr Jones thinks that the trekking will accelerate the arthritis and that Grace will return with swollen and painful knees which may take months to settle down to their present state. The trip may increase the likelihood of Grace needing early knee replacements. From a medical point of view, trekking will be harmful to Grace's musculo–skeletal health. Dr Jones explains this to Grace who then goes away to think it over. Later she tells Dr Jones that she will be going trekking, as this has been one of her goals for many years and she thinks this is her last opportunity. She understands that her knees will suffer, but thinks the overall value and meaning of the trip are worth any subsequent ill effects.

In this scenario, Grace has sought medical advice to help her make a decision with health implications. She accepted the prediction that her knees will be harmed, but decided to go ahead with the trip. We might not have made the same decision in her place, but we can understand her right to make this decision, and we can recognize that this is very much her decision, based upon a thoughtful consideration of the risks and benefits to her. In ethical terms, we describe decisions like this as autonomous, reflecting the wishes and values of the person involved and in some important way, belonging to that person rather than being imposed by an external force.

What is autonomy and why is it important?

Autonomy can be a tricky term to define or understand. We can describe people, decisions, or actions as autonomous. An autonomous person shapes and directs his or her own life, based upon their own values, to bring about their own choices and plans (Young 2001). Autonomous actions or decisions reflect a person's full understanding and evaluation of the relevant issues, taking place in a voluntary way without any coercion or manipulation. The idea of free action, not being coerced or forced by anyone else, is central to understanding autonomy.

Much of our thinking about autonomy has been influenced by J.S. Mill. Why did Mill think that personal autonomy is so important? Is it because autonomy is valuable for itself, or because things are likely to turn out better if people are left alone to make their own decisions?

Box 6.1 The liberty principle

"Over himself, over his own body and mind, the individual is sovereign."

Exception to the principle

"The only purpose for which power can be rightfully exercised over any member of a civilised community, against his will, is to prevent harm to others. His own good, either physical or moral, is not a sufficient warrant." (Mill 1991, p. 14)

The second set of reasons are straightforward to understand: things are likely to turn out better if people make their own decisions because:

(a) Individuals are the best placed to know and understand what is important to them—they are the best judge of their own interests.

(b) Individuals are more likely than anyone else to be motivated to try and get what is best for themselves.

(c) People resent interference, even well meaning interference, so it may be counterproductive to force people into a course of action even if it is for their own good.

As well as these consequentialist reasons, autonomy is important for itself, because being autonomous expresses aspects of being human that we value highly, like the capacity to make decisions which reflect our uniqueness as individuals, and the capacity to develop in ways that foster our particular character traits and interests. Without the freedom to be autonomous, we would lose much of our individuality (Christie and Hoffmaster 1986; Kultgen 1995).

Autonomy in practice

In ethical terms, we recognize the importance of personal autonomy through the obligation that doctors have to respect the autonomy of patients. The principle of respect for patients' autonomy protects the right that patients have to control their own bodies and to make their own decisions about medical treatment. Respecting patient autonomy means that doctors should not examine patients or give treatments unless the patient has given their informed consent for this to happen.

Historically speaking, the idea that patients should be autonomous with regard to their medical care is a relatively recent phenomenon, emerging from the 1960s in the wake of civil rights movements. As discussed in Chapter 4, the idea that doctors are experts because of their medical knowledge runs deep, and this expertise is often used as a justification for doctors to make decisions for patients. As well as historical precedent, there are practical reasons for thinking that patients either may not want to or be able to make their own decisions about medical care, for various reasons. Despite these reservations, the principle of respect for patient autonomy has become one of the central planks of contemporary medical ethics, with the practice of informed consent serving as a legal reminder of its importance. Later in the chapter we will look at some of the practicalities and implications for the doctor–patient relationship of the duty to respect patient autonomy.

Before discussing informed consent in detail, it is worth considering what we mean by 'respect'. How can doctors show that they respect the right of their patients to make their own decisions, even if they disagree with the decision? Respecting another person involves recognizing that that person has a unique nature with their own feelings and desires, and the capacity to work out what is best for themselves (Downie and Calman 1994). Respect also involves practical aspects, such as maintaining confidentiality (see Chapter 3) and protecting patient privacy, as well as using a courteous manner and addressing people in their preferred way. The process of respecting is important; in the scenario at the beginning of the chapter we did not spell out how Dr Jones actually replied to Grace's enquiry. She may have explained her prognosis in a sympathetic way that expressed her understanding of the importance of the trip and the need for Grace to have as much information as possible to make her decision. Or Dr Jones may have responded in a bullying way, implying that trekking was a ridiculous idea and that Grace would need extra medical care as a result. Respect requires us to understand the impact both of what we are saying and the way we are saying it, avoiding patronizing or judgemental assumptions.

Informed consent

Informed consent is a mechanism for people to control what happens to them, forming an important part of respecting autonomy. The main aim of informed consent is to ensure that people are acting freely, without coercion or deception (O'Neill 2003). Informed consent is the process through which people can authorize what happens to them or who touches them, making medical treatments morally acceptable. The law strongly upholds this moral position; before you can examine, treat, or care for a competent adult person, you must obtain their informed consent (DOH 2002). Without consent, touching a patient or taking blood is potential battery, even if the action is intended to help rather than harm the patient (Mason and McCall Smith 1999).

In general practice, consent is often taken for granted. There are no forms to sign as for surgery, and patients are usually considered to consent to their care by the fact of turning up. But this does not decrease the moral importance of making sure that the conditions for informed consent are met. How can we tell when or if consent is informed? The conditions for informed consent try to ensure that any decision the patient has made is autonomous by asking three questions:

(a) Is this person competent to make the decision?

(b) Do they understand the necessary information?

(c) Are they making the decision freely?

Competence

Competence is to do with the ability of a person to make decisions that reflect their values and their concern for their own well-being, or in other words, their *capacity* to make autonomous decisions (Young 2001). How can we tell if a person is competent to make a decision, especially if it is one that we have difficulty understanding?

Case 6.2

Paul McKinney is a 34-year-old patient with schizophrenia. He takes long-acting psychotropic medication for his schizophrenia which has been well controlled for the past few months, with the exception of some fixed paranoid delusions about the media. Dr Jeremy Chu is called to do a house visit because Paul has had

---

Case 6.2 *(Cont.)*

24 hours of severe abdominal pain. On examination, Paul is febrile and has the clinical signs of appendicitis. Dr Chu explains the diagnosis in terms of part of the bowel being infected, with the risk of rupturing, and the possible consequences if this occurs. He recommends to Paul that he go straight to the local emergency department for observation and possible operation. Paul seems to understand what Dr Chu is saying, and the risks of not going to hospital, but he says that he will not go to the hospital because he dislikes the way that they treat him there, he does not want an operation, and he wants to see if he can recover with treatment from Dr Chu.

Is this a competent decision? Dr Chu is in a difficult position, as he thinks it is very much in Paul's best interests to go to the hospital, but at the same time, Paul seems to understand the risks. Paul fulfils the legal criteria for competence, or capacity to consent to or refuse treatment.

Box 6.2 Criteria for capacity to consent to or refuse treatment

1 Does the person understand the nature, purpose, and effects of the proposed treatment?

2 Is the patient able to comprehend and retain relevant information?

3 Has the patient believed the information and weighed it in the balance with other considerations when making their choice? (Mason and McCall Smith 1999, p. 263.)

Unlike the decision made by Grace in the first example, it is much harder to understand Paul's decision. A dislike of hospitals hardly seems a good enough reason to refuse potentially life-saving treatment. Yet as long as Paul's decision is competent, it does not matter how irrational or wrong it seems to others; there is no moral or legal basis for compelling him to go to hospital. Difficult though it may be, Dr Chu has to accept Paul's decision, as well as ongoing responsibility for Paul's medical care, guided by the interventions that he will accept.

Despite Paul's schizophrenia, he is competent to make this decision about treatment for appendicitis as he can understand the nature of appendicitis and the likely consequences of his decision, and he has weighed up this information against his reasons for not wishing to go to hospital. Competence is assessed relative to the decision at hand.

Case 6.2 continued

With Paul's consent, Dr Chu discusses Paul's condition with the surgical registrar and treats him with a stat dose of iv antibiotics. When he visits the next morning, Paul is worse, with obvious dehydration and signs of peritonitis. Dr Chu once again explains what has happened and stresses that without fluid replacement and further antibiotics, Paul is at risk of dying.

This time Paul agrees to admission.

We tend to think of consent as a one-off event, either the patient refuses or consents to treatment. However, patients have a right to review their decision and alter it, in the light of changing circumstances. We may not know why Paul changed his mind, but Dr Chu had an obligation to keep checking Paul's decision, and to keep the channels of communication open in case he revised his decision. The ongoing nature of consent is important, people's views about a treatment may well change after they have experienced for themselves the side-effects and benefits over time.

Understanding

One of the conditions for autonomous decisions is that the person concerned understands the full implications of their decision. This is perhaps the hardest condition to come to grips with—how much information does a patient need to understand fully the possible consequences of their decision, and how can a doctor make sure that the patient is both informed and understands this information?

To understand in the medical situation, the patient needs to actually comprehend the language used by the doctor and then be able to relate that information to their own circumstances. How do we judge whether or not understanding has been achieved? From the patient's perspective, the language of medicine is often foreign and difficult to interpret in terms of knowing what is significant and what is not. In the process of becoming a doctor, a person doubles his or her vocabulary (Rogers 1992). This means that a large proportion of the words doctors use are unfamiliar to the general population.

A certain amount of knowledge is necessary before a patient can understand the relevance of what is being said. A patient may feel that they have enough information to make a decision, but it is probably only in retrospect that they can properly judge whether or not they had understood what their treatment would be like. Research suggests that when people are asked in retrospect about the information they were given, up to 40% of patients do not understand the nature and purpose of their treatment and 45% can not recall any major risks or complications (Cassileth *et al.* 1980; Olver *et al.* 1994).

One problem with understanding is the difference between understanding what will happen, and actually knowing what that will feel like. A side-effect of nocturnal diuresis affecting 30–40% of people who take a particular drug may sound acceptable to a patient, but after three weeks of interrupted sleep, the patient may realize that this is unacceptable to them.

Another problem with understanding is the inherently uncertain nature of medicine. Despite their best efforts, doctors are not able to accurately predict what will happen in each case. If a person suffers a rare side-effect from treatment, although they may have been aware that this was possible, it is not clear that this is the same as understanding that it might actually happen to them, and what it would be like if it did happen.

Case 6.3

Robert Williamson is a 56-year-old man, who visits Dr Bowler fairly infrequently. One day he comes in to see Dr Bowler requesting a test for prostate cancer. His uncle has just been diagnosed with disseminated prostate cancer, and Robert Williamson wants a test to make sure that the same thing does not happen to him.

How much information will Robert need to make an informed decision about the PSA test, and how well can he understand the potential risks of the situation while he is distressed about his uncle and clinging to the belief that the test is necessary to 'prevent him from getting cancer'? Dr Bowler needs time to explain the nature of screening tests, and the difference between screening and prevention. Robert cannot give his informed consent for the test until he understands the benefits and potential harms. Sometimes it seems easier and quicker to do the test rather than explain all the pros and cons to the patient, but adopting this course of action ignores the moral obligation to respect the autonomy of patients. We know that patients have a strong desire for information (Ende *et al.* 1989; Ong *et al.* 1995; Charles *et al.* 1997) and that doctors consistently underestimate this (Sullivan *et al.* 2001).

In the UK, there are no set rules for judging how much information a doctor should give a patient. From a moral point of view, the aim is to try to ensure that the patient has all of the information that they need to make an autonomous decision, which means tailoring the information to the interests and concerns of that patient. This is a demanding requirement, and one that is time-consuming to fulfil. However, in general practice, it may be easier to reach this standard than in branches of secondary or tertiary care, as general practice allows an ongoing relationship in which information may be exchanged over time, and in which the GP may know the patient well enough to be able to 'fit' the information to the patient in a meaningful way. Patients in general practice can come to know their GP's communication style, and to trust that the GP knows them well enough to explain the important and relevant information and omit the rest.

From a legal point of view, a doctor who does not give the patient enough information may be considered negligent. The UK law uses a professional standard to judge negligence. This means that your practice (i.e. the information that you tell the patient) has to be within the boundaries of acceptable practice (i.e. what at least some doctors usually tell patients) as judged by a responsible body of medical opinion. This is known as the Bolam ruling or standard (Mason and McCall Smith 1999). However, the courts recognize the importance of doctors disclosing *all* risks that may be relevant to that specific patient, irrespective of usual professional practice. This means using the patient's perspective rather than that of the medical profession. This standard is known as the prudent patient standard, and is ethically preferable to the professional standard, as this is more likely to help the patient to make a fully informed decision. The prudent patient standard operates in other jurisdictions, such as Australia, and it may only be a matter of time before it becomes legally accepted in the UK. (See below for a discussion of withholding or manipulating information.)

Voluntariness

The final condition for autonomous decisions is voluntariness; to be autonomous, a person's decision should not be manipulated or coerced in any way, by a health professional, by relatives, or anyone else.

Case 6.4

Mrs Butler is an elderly woman who lives alone, with weekly visits from her daughter. One day her daughter Alice makes an appointment for Mrs Butler to see her GP, Dr Shah. In the consultation, Alice says that her mother has not been well lately. She has no appetite and has lost weight. Alice would like Dr Shah to examine Mrs Butler and do some tests, to find out what is wrong. Mrs Butler is silent for most of the consultation, and when asked if she is willing to have an examination, her daughter answers, "Of course".

During the examination, Dr Shah asks Alice to leave the room. Mrs Butler has a large craggy mass in her left breast, and an enlarged liver. Dr Shah tells Mrs Butler that there is something wrong in her breast and says that she would need to do some tests to find out exactly what it is, but that it may be cancer. She asks if she is willing to have the tests. At this stage Alice comes back into the room, wanting to know what the examination has shown and what tests Dr Shah is going to do. Dr Shah again asks Alice to leave the room, but she insists that her mother wants her there, appealing to Mrs Butler for confirmation. Mrs Butler nods her head and asks the doctor to explain things to Alice. Dr Shah outlines the situation and Alice says, "Of course Mum wants the tests, when can they be done?"

Dr Shah is worried that Alice is coercing Mrs Butler into this consultation and the investigations, and that she does not know what Mrs Butler would really like to happen.

Discussions about autonomy can give the impression that it is easy to distinguish between a decision that is voluntary and one that is coerced in some way, but in reality, the distinction can be tricky. From the information in this scenario, Mrs Butler appears to be pressured, if not bullied, by her daughter. For Dr Shah, the task is to find out Mrs Butler's own preferences, starting with her knowledge of Mrs Butler based upon their existing relationship. Maybe Mrs Butler always looks to her daughter for guidance, and most of her medical care happens through the agency of the daughter. On the other hand, maybe Mrs Butler has mentioned in previous consultations that if she gets a potentially terminal illness, she would not want to have any treatment, or that she finds her daughter over-interfering. Dr Shah cannot be sure of Mrs Butler's own preferences about investigation and treatment until she has had a chance to talk to her on her own. Arranging this may involve some subterfuge on her part, but it is essential to find out this information.

This case raises a wider point about the decisions that people make; we have said that to be autonomous a decision must in some way belong to that person, to be in character rather than be directed by another. However, humans are social creatures, living in relationships with others whose views we respect and whose advice we seek, especially when we need to make serious decisions. People *are* influenced by the wishes and desires of others, and responding to those influences strengthens and deepens our relationships. Does this somehow limit or damage personal autonomy? If we consider that having meaningful relationships is an important part of what people wish for themselves, then we have to look at autonomy in a broader sense than that of purely individualistic decision-making. If people are free to choose their relationships, then accepting advice and being influenced within those freely chosen relationships may not compromise autonomy at all. Relationships contribute to who people are, so that part of being 'in character' is to make decisions with input from others, in the context of significant relationships.

How can we accept this view of autonomy without losing the requirement for voluntariness? We need to consider the context of decision-making, and the relationship between the person making the decision and those around them. Cases at either end of the spectrum will be easy to identify: for example a woman brought to the GP by an overbearing partner for a referral for tubal ligation that she does not want is being coerced in an unacceptable way. On the other hand, an elderly parent brought for a check up by a concerned son in a way that reflects the long-standing dynamics of their relationship can be an example of acceptable influence and persuasion.

Doctors have a responsibility to use all available information to work out what is going on in each situation, asking questions like:

(a) Why does this patient have her relative with her?

(b) Is this the decision that I would have expected in this situation?

(c) Whose interests are being met by this decision?

(d) Does the patient seem comfortable with this choice?

Any pre-existing doctor–patient relationship is an invaluable resource, especially if the GP knows what kinds of things the patient usually trusts him to do.

Is illness itself coercive? In some sense it is, as when we are ill we do all sorts of things that we would prefer not to, like having blood tests or taking medication. But although illness narrows our range of choices, illness itself is not considered coercive in the same way that actions taken by other human beings may be. Illness happens by chance, making it morally neutral. We cannot rationally blame someone else for making us ill, in the same way that we could blame someone who coerced us by holding a gun to our head. Human actions and their consequences can be judged on a moral scale, but events like illness that occur irrespective of human action cannot be judged on the same scale (leaving aside events such as bio-terrorism or intentional exposure to infectious diseases).

Doctors and other health professionals can be sources of manipulation or undue persuasion, either consciously or unconsciously. In theory, voluntary informed consent involves the patient making a selection between alternative courses of action, having received information about these from a doctor. The doctor should present relevant information in a neutral manner so that the patient can choose the best option for them rather than being influenced by the preferences of the doctor. However, it can be difficult for doctors to present information in an entirely neutral manner. Often the doctor does think that one course of action is better than another, and it may be hard to conceal this view. The way the information is presented can have a significant effect on the patient's view about a treatment. Usually we describe the benefits of a proposed course of treatment, before describing the side-effects or complications. This encourages an initial commitment to the treatment before the full extent of any disadvantages are apparent (Cialdini *et al.* 1978; Faden and Beauchamp 1986). Once the psychological commitment has been made, people are less likely to withdraw their consent even when faced with quite significant drawbacks. Is this a form of acceptable persuasion, or unacceptable manipulation?

It is important to keep sight of any motives the doctor has for suggesting one particular course of action over another; strong persuasion or unintentional manipulation motivated by beneficence is more acceptable than actions motivated by, for example, personal gain (such as persuading a patient to enter a drug trial so that the GP will receive payment). Patients attend GPs for medical advice and treatment, providing some prima facie justification for GPs to put the medical case quite strongly, within the bounds of avoiding deception and answering questions truthfully. Patients who disagree with the medical model of illness and its associated values are free to seek health care from alternative and complementary practitioners (within the limits of their personal resources). However, doctors may be influenced by other factors such as religious beliefs that are not necessarily known to patients, and who may find them unwelcome. For example a GP with a strong belief in the sanctity of life may believe it is wrong to refer a woman for a termination of pregnancy, and do his best to dissuade her. In situations where GPs' personal beliefs influence their clinical decisions, GPs have an obligation to make their beliefs explicit, or to refer the patient to another practitioner.

One reason for withholding information is the fear of self-fulfilling prophecies, for example with regard to side-effects (Christie and Hoffmaster 1986). If a patient who has just been prescribed beta-blockers for example, is told that one of the side-effects is tiredness, this may create the expectation in that patient that they will feel tired. This is a bit like the placebo effect, but instead of feeling better because that is what is expected, the patient experiences the side-effect because this is what they are expecting. Is there an ethical way to minimize the placebo effect for side-effects? Different GPs have different ways of explaining side-effects, and patients have varying desires for information, making it hard to generalize. One option is to review the patient at an early time and ask if they have experienced any side-effects, leaving it up to the patient to identify any unusual or new effects which the GP may then confirm. However, this can leave the patient not knowing what to expect and potentially distressed by seemingly unexplained symptoms. Decisions as to how much information about side-effects to tell patients require judgement, based upon the GP's knowledge of the patient and the frequency and severity of the possible side-effects. If a patient asks about the nature of any possible side-effects, the doctor is obliged to respond honestly.

There are also pragmatic reasons why GPs might withhold information, the most obvious being lack of time (Christie and Hoffmaster 1986). This is a constant pressure, trying to meet the needs of individual patients for information while also meeting overall patient demand. (See also Chapter 5.) In Chapter 2 we discussed the importance of trust in the doctor–patient relationship, and it is worth referring back to this in the context of giving information to patients, to pose the question: "What does this patient trust me to do, and how much am I expecting them to trust my judgement in this case?" In a patient–doctor relationship characterized by trust, it is possible to develop mutual short cuts, for example the patient might ask: "Is there anything that you think I should know about this treatment?", trusting the GP to tailor information to their specific circumstances. Conversely, GPs need a certain amount of trust in their patients to provide enough information for patients to make informed choices. Trust smoothes the process for patients to have some control over decision-making.

Another reason why GPs might withhold information is because of discomfort over the issues that might be raised. This typically occurs in relation to disclosing bad news about poor prognoses, when the GP might be faced with discussing the impending death of the patient. (See Chapter 8 for specific discussion of end of life issues.) Recent research from the US indicates a significant gap between patients' desire for information about serious diagnoses and physicians' estimates of these. Only 42% of physicians said patients want to be told all details about a serious illness. Fifty-seven per cent said patients want to be told only in general terms and 1% said patients want no information. However up to 82% of patients wanted to be told all the details, with this figure dropping to 61% for patients over 60 years of age (Sullivan *et al.* 2001). GPs may feel uncomfortable breaking bad news and discussing death, but this is not a morally acceptable reason for withholding information.

Discussions about informed consent can become side-tracked into concerns over the extent of information to be disclosed, or how much persuasion is acceptable, and whether or not the patient is making the decision. At times it is worth standing back to remember the ethical point at stake which is that it is wrong to deceive or coerce people, as this prevents them from making autonomous choices. Information is a means to this: if a patient receives explanations so that she is able to understand the implications of accepting or refusing a treatment, she is then in a position to make a choice if she wishes to. The obligation of doctors is to promote or protect the capacity of the patient for autonomous action by providing enough information so that the patient has the opportunity to make a meaningful decision.

Limits on autonomy and difficult cases

Case 6.5

Elsie Butterworth is a 68-year-old woman with alcoholism. She drinks to dangerous levels, has had a number of serious falls, and is likely to die from her disease. Dr Whittaker has seen Elsie on numerous occasions and each time informs her of the dangers of her current levels of drinking and the need to undergo some kind of rehabilitation. Elsie acknowledges the dangers and seems to agree that she should do something about her drinking, but each time she fails to keep appointments and her drinking does not diminish. Dr Whittaker thinks that Elsie is not acting autonomously, because of her alcohol addiction. It would be in her best interests to receive treatment, but Dr Whittaker is not able to admit Elsie for compulsory treatment as alcoholism and drug addiction are specifically excluded by section 1 (3) of the Mental Health Act.

GPs are often faced with patients who do not seem autonomous due to addiction or psychological disorders, but who cannot receive compulsory treatment based upon their best interests, because they do not meet the criteria for compulsory treatment under the Mental Health Act. How can the GP fulfil his ethical obligations in these situations?

The Mental Health Act tries to strike a balance between protecting people who are incapacitated by mental illness, and at the same time, protecting the rights of people to refuse unwanted treatment. This is always going to be a difficult balance that leaves some patients who are not able to make autonomous decisions, perhaps due to psychological compulsions, outside the jurisdiction of the Act. For GPs the task can seem both endless and thankless, fruitlessly repeating the same advice, with the same lack of effect while the patient becomes worse. It is important to recognize the GP's lack of agency in these situations; GPs do not have the power to intervene in terms of compulsory treatment for the patient's good except in very limited circumstances (see below). Acknowledgement that changing the situation is beyond the control of the GP can help to ease frustration and open the way for looking at ethical responses. The GP has ongoing obligations to maintain a respectful relationship with the patient and to offer such care as the patient is able or willing to accept. Building up a relationship may eventually lead to change for the patient, but at the very least, an ongoing relationship offers the best chance of minimizing further harm to the patient.

Sometimes it is possible to develop creative solutions with patients, protecting long-term patient autonomy through periods of diminished capacity.

Case 6.6

Ian Johnson is a 32-year-old lawyer with established bi-polar disease. When he becomes manic, he is very articulate and persuasive, and it has been very difficult to admit him for compulsory treatment. He has had prolonged periods of mania during which he refused treatment. This has led to serious consequences for his personal life, employment, and financial security. After one episode of mania, he asked his GP, Dr McDonald to help him to avoid similar situations in the future. Ian arranged an advance directive that authorizes Dr McDonald to arrange compulsory treatment irrespective of anything that he might say or do at the time.

This kind of arrangement demonstrates the value of a trusting doctor–patient relationship. Ian is able to transfer decision-making power to Dr McDonald because he trusts that Dr McDonald will act in his best interests at a time when, because of his illness, he is not autonomous. Ian's long-term autonomy is protected; his autonomous decision, made when he is well, is to be treated for his illness. Handing over power is a way of protecting his long-term interests. Dr McDonald is able to intervene earlier in the illness than would otherwise be possible, and to use the directive to override any illness-fuelled resistance from Ian.

This example used a formal mechanism for transferring decision-making power from the patient to the GP, however less formal examples are common in practice. Patients who are usually thoughtful and decisive may want their GP to make decisions about treatment when they are acutely unwell. For example a woman who has made informed decisions about contraception and screening may ask the GP to do whatever he or she thinks necessary when she is febrile and vomiting with pyelonephritis. Taking control in this way does not infringe the autonomy of the patient, because it is at the request of the patient.

Treating without consent

Sometimes it is not possible to inform a patient about their illness and proposed management, or to seek consent from them. The patient may be unconscious, incompetent due to a psychiatric illness or mental disability, or have limited understanding, such as in the case of a child. If treatment is given without consent, this is known as non-voluntary treatment, and must be based upon the best interests of the patient. In general, treatment should be aimed at minimizing harm and restoring the patient's health as far as possible. Interventions should be limited to the least invasive consistent with those goals. If possible, definitive or irreversible treatment should be deferred until the patient regains (or in the case of a child, reaches) competence. In England and Wales, no one else can give consent for an incompetent or unconscious adult. The situation is different in Scotland under the *Adults with Incapacity (Scotland) Act 2000* which provides for the appointment of welfare guardians or attorneys with the power to consent to treatment on behalf of the nominated person.

Box 6.3 Treating without consent

Non-voluntary treatment: treatment without consent because patient unable either to give or withhold consent.

Involuntary treatment: consent withheld by patient, but treatment given involuntarily under the Mental Health Act 1983.

In life-threatening emergencies the situation is usually straightforward; unless the GP has any reason to believe that the patient would not want to be treated in these circumstances, it is ethically required and legally acceptable to provide emergency treatment, aimed at saving the person's life and returning them as soon as possible to a conscious state.

Patients with mental impairment may receive involuntary treatment if this is in their best interests. Who should judge this? Usually the law permits medical practitioners to have the final say as to whether or not a medical treatment is in the interests of a patient, but any assessment of interests should include information from friends and relatives, and take into account the patient's known values and any previously expressed wishes. Although relatives or friends cannot give consent for an incompetent patient, they are an invaluable source of information for the doctor who is trying to work out the likely benefit to a patient of a proposed treatment.

Adults who are incompetent due to mental disorders may be admitted to hospital as involuntary patients either as an emergency, for assessment, or for treatment under the Mental Health Act 1983. The conditions covered by these three forms of admission vary, but the intent is to limit involuntary admission to those who are not competent, by virtue of their mental disorder, to make autonomous decisions (Mason and McCall Smith 1999). Patients with psychiatric illness can only be given compulsory treatment for their psychiatric illness, not for any concomitant physical illness. This recognizes the fact that even though a patient may be incompetent for some decisions, this does not mean that they are incompetent for all decisions.

The third group of patients who might require treatment without consent are children. Parents are able to refuse or consent to treatment for their children when that child is not considered competent. If the child is considered competent by the doctor, in terms of being able to understand the proposed treatment, alternatives, and consequences, then the child has the right to consent to treatment, irrespective of the views of the parents. (This point is fully discussed under Gillick competence in Chapter 7.)

External limits on autonomy

Much of our discussion in this chapter has focused on autonomy as a personal capacity or condition for decisions and actions. This approach ignores the wider social context and the ways that choices are framed and directed by external forces. First of all, autonomous choices may be limited by the circumstances of the patient. A patient may prefer physiotherapy to a steroid injection for a shoulder problem, but it may be impossible for them to attend a series of physiotherapy sessions due to child care responsibilities or difficulties in taking time off from work. A treatment may be too expensive, or travelling to the place where it is provided may be too difficult. Patients have many different factors to consider when making decisions, so that personal circumstances can have the effect of directing or limiting choices (Rogers 1999). These can include the attitudes and beliefs of families and friends, and the kind of opportunities that are available in particular social settings, as well as more concrete factors like cost.

Public resources may be limited, so that a patient's preferred choice of treatment is not available, either at all or in their area. Lack of resources, or restrictions on existing facilities are constant themes in the NHS. The provision of new NHS interventions is now under the control of the National Institute for Clinical Excellence, with the aim of ensuring uniform provision of approved interventions, but there is little monitoring of the flow-on effects of these decisions. The mandated introduction of a new intervention may lead to curtailing other services in the context of fixed budgets, with variable effects upon the options available to patients.

The range of options available in the treatment of any problem has been influenced and shaped by circumstances beyond the control of either patient or GP (Rogers 2002). The current interest in evidence-based medicine has led to the promotion of interventions judged to be effective by the standards of EBM; but the research programmes which provide data for EBM reflect professional and commercial interests, rather than those of patients. This means that the range of options open to the patient may not include those that she would prefer (Sherwin 1992). The patient may be presented with a choice between pharmacological and surgical treatment for a problem and be free to choose between those options. However an alternative approach to treatment, for example by dietary manipulation, meditation, or exercise may not be offered as an option due to a lack of high quality information about such options.

At a wider lever, people's desires and choices are shaped by the society they live in, so that although apparently free to make choices, our ideas about many issues, which feel like our own ideas, reflect widely held values in our society. For example, a woman may be apparently free to accept or reject antenatal screening or cosmetic surgery, but if the prevailing social norms are to do everything possible to have a perfect baby or a particular physical appearance, we may question the sense in which decisions about these matters are autonomous (Sherwin 1992).

Autonomy and responsibility

In this chapter we have outlined an account of patient autonomy and emphasized the importance of providing information and avoiding manipulation or coercion of patients. What are the implications of this account for responsibility within the consultation? Must patients, to be autonomous, make their own decisions at all times? Who is then responsible for medical care?

First of all it is important to make the distinction between being well informed and making choices. Respect for patient autonomy requires that GPs provide patients with enough information so that they can understand what is wrong and what might be done about it, unless the patient has clearly indicated that they prefer not to have this information. The responsibility for this lies with GPs. As discussed above, research shows that patients consistently indicate a strong desire for information about their medical problems (Ende *et al*. 1989; Ong *et al*. 1995; Charles *et al*. 1997). This does not always translate directly into a preference for decision-making. Research including studies based in primary care have found that the majority of patients preferred their doctors to make decisions (Ende *et al*. 1989; Ong *et al*. 1995; Bradley *et al*. 1996). In general it is a minority of patients who prefer to make their own decisions, although this may change over time as patient expectations change. This leaves much responsibility and control over decision-making with doctors, but in a non-coercive way as this is with permission from patients. However, this permission cannot be assumed but requires constant checking to make sure that this patient, in this consultation, prefers to take medical advice rather than make their own decision. Much of the time patients agree with medical advice, so that a decision about management emerges from the consultation rather than taking the form of a formal and discrete decision.

Does this leave patients with little responsibility within the doctor–patient relationship? This topic is explored more fully in Chapter 4, but it is worth repeating here that although patients do have responsibilities, the greater responsibilities lie with the doctor. This can create problems, for example in determining who is responsible for ensuring that patients receive results from investigations.

Case 6.7

Matthew Slyth came to see Dr Carter with abdominal pain. After taking a history and examination, Dr Carter referred Matthew for gastroscopy, with clear instructions to telephone for the results if he had not heard from the Hackney Road Practice within 10 days. In the meantime, Dr Carter went on annual leave. The gastroscopy result came back to the practice, and, in Dr Carter's absence, was given to Dr Chu, who entered the result onto the computer. The report was then filed in Matthew's notes. Dr Carter did his paperwork upon his return from holiday, but as the report did not appear there, forgot about it. Matthew did not telephone for his results at any stage. One year later, Matthew presented with melena from an untreated gastric ulcer which had been identified by the gastroscopy. He made a formal complaint that he had not been given the gastroscopy result.

Transmitting results to patients can be fraught with pitfalls. Posting results or telephoning patients may breach confidentiality, but leaving patients to follow-up may have disastrous consequences, as in Case 6.7. Did the patient in this case have a responsibility to ring for his results? If this is the arrangement agreed between GP and patient, then surely he had a moral responsibility to do so (although the legal responsibility lies with the doctor). If a patient does not ring for results, the GP is left wondering if this is because he or she does not want them, which may be an autonomous refusal of information, or merely due to a slip of memory. Given the fallibility of human memory and the difficulty of eliminating all administrative mistakes from practice, joint responsibility is probably the safest method.

Conclusion

In this chapter we have looked at the important ethical duty that doctors have to respect the autonomy of patients. This duty requires GPs to support patients in making voluntary informed decisions. We have discussed competence, understanding, and voluntariness in relation to autonomy and informed consent, and looked at the situation for patients who are not able to give consent. Difficult issues concerning autonomy arise in relation to patients who are incompetent, or who are unable to act autonomously for other reasons. Sometimes the constraints on patient autonomy are external, arising from the circumstances in which people live. Finally we have looked at responsibility for medical decisions.

References

Bradley, J., Zia, M., and Hamilton, N. (1996). Patient preferences for control in medical decision making: a scenario-based approach. *Family Medicine* **28** (7), 496–501.

Cassileth, B., Zupkis, R., Sutton-Smith, K., and March, V. (1980). Informed consent: Why are its goals imperfectly realised? *New England Journal of Medicine* **302** (16), 896–900.

Charles, C., Gafni, A., and Whelan, T. (1997). Shared decision-making in the medical encounter: What does it mean? (Or it takes at least two to tango.) *Social Science and Medicine* **44** (5), 681–92.

Christie, R. and Hoffmaster, B. (1986). *Ethical issues in family medicine.* Oxford University Press, New York, NY.

Cialdini, R.B., Cacioppo, J.T., Bassett, R., and Miller, J.A. (1978). Low-ball procedure for producing compliance: commitment then cost. *Journal of Personality and Social Psychology* **36** (5), 463–76.

Department of Health. (2002). *Consent guidance.* http://www.doh.gov.uk/consent/guidance.htm

Downie, R. and Calman, K. (1994). *Healthy respect: ethics in health care,* (2nd edn). Oxford University Press, Oxford.

Ende, J., Kazis, L., Ash, A., and Moskowitz, M. (1989). Measuring patients' desire for autonomy. *Journal of General Internal Medicine* **4** (Jan/Feb), 23–30.

Faden, R.R. and Beauchamp, T.L. (1986). *A history and theory of informed consent.* Oxford University Press, New York, NY.

Kultgen, J. (1995). *Autonomy and intervention: parentalism in the caring life.* Oxford University Press, New York, NY.

Mason, J. and McCall Smith, R. (1999). *Law and medical ethics,* (5th edn). Butterworths, London.

Mill, J.S. (1991). In Gray J. (ed.) *On liberty and other essays.* Oxford University Press, Oxford.

Olver, I., Turrell, S., Olszewski, N., and Willson, K. (1994) The impact of a full disclosure information and consent form on patients receiving standard cytotoxic chemotherapy. *Proceedings,* Australian Bioethics Association Third National Conference.

O'Neill, O. (2003). Some limits of informed consent. *Journal of Medical Ethics* **29**, 4–7.

Ong, L., de Haes, J., Hoos, A., and Lammes, F. (1995). Doctor–patient communication: a review of the literature. *Social Science and Medicine* **40** (7), 903–18.

Rogers, A.W. (1992). *Textbook of anatomy.* Churchill Livingstone, Edinburgh.

Rogers, W.A. (1999). Beneficence in general practice: an empirical investigation. *Journal of Medical Ethics* **25** (5), 388–93.

Rogers, W.A. (2002). Evidence-based medicine in practice: limiting or facilitating patient choice? *Health Expectations* **5**, 95–103.

Sherwin, S. (1992). *No longer patient.* Temple University Press, Philadelphia, PA.

Sullivan, R., Menapace, L., and White, R. (2001). Truth-telling and patient diagnoses. *Journal of Medical Ethics* **27**, 192–7.

Young, R. (2001). Informed consent and patient autonomy. In Kuhse, H. and Singer, P. (ed.) *A companion to bioethics,* pp. 441–51. Blackwell Publishers, Oxford.

Further reading

Charles, C., Gafni, A., and Whelan, T. (1997). Shared decision-making in the medical encounter: what does it mean? (Or it takes at least two to tango). *Social Science and Medicine* **44** (5), 681–692.

Department of Health (2002). *Consent.* http://www.doh.gov.uk/consent/

General Medical Council. (1998). *Seeking patient's consent: the ethical considerations*. General Medical Council, London. *http://www.gmc-uk.org/ standards/defaults.htm*

Journal of Medical Ethics (2003). **29**, 2–40. *Symposium on consent and confidentiality*. Series of eleven articles on various aspects of consent and confidentiality.

Quill, T.E. and Brody, H. (1996). Physician recommendations and patient autonomy: finding a balance between physician power and patient choice. *Annals of Internal Medicine* **125**, 763–69.

Rogers, W.A. (2002). Evidence-based medicine in practice: Limiting or facilitating patient choice? *Health Expectations* **5**, 95–103.

Rogers, W.A. (2002). Whose autonomy? Which choice? A study of general practitioners' attitudes towards patient autonomy in the management of low back pain. *Family Practice* **19**, 140–5.

Chapter 7

Ethical issues at the beginning of life

Introduction

In many ways, consultations to do with pregnancy and childbirth can provide some of the most rewarding moments in general practice. Confirming a highly desired pregnancy for a woman or attending the delivery of a healthy baby are times when GPs are able to share in the happiness of patients, privileged by virtue of being a GP to attend at these occasions, but relieved of the need for any medical action, because all is going well. On the other hand, issues such as abortion and assisted fertility techniques raise a host of ethical questions. Although GPs do not directly provide these services, they are often involved as the first point of contact, with responsibilities for discussing options with patients and referring onto other services. In this chapter, we look at ethical issues in relation to providing contraception, responding to requests for abortions and for referral to reproductive technologies, providing antenatal care, and caring for women during labour and delivery.

Contraception

Case 7.1

Lucy, a 13-year-old girl, comes to see her GP, Dr Fiona McDonald. Dr McDonald has known Lucy from childhood, and she has cared for all members of her family. Lucy has never attended on her own before and seems quite nervous. Eventually she says that she would like to go on the pill, to make her periods regular. After some discussion, Lucy explains that she has a 15-year-old boyfriend and that they are planning to have sex, but that she is very worried about the possibility of pregnancy. She has read about contraception in magazines and thinks that she would prefer the certainty and 'lack of fuss' of the pill compared with barrier methods. Lucy is worried that her mother, whom she describes as 'overprotective', would be thrown into a panic if she learnt about Lucy's intentions. She asks Dr McDonald for a prescription, and for assurance that she will not reveal her request to anyone.

Access to safe reliable contraception is necessary for women to avoid the possible consequences of unwanted pregnancies. Without such access, other important aspects of women's lives such as education, employment, or relationships can be jeopardized. The majority of consultations for advice and information about contraception are very straightforward; once a women is well informed about the possible options, she is able to make up her own mind as to which method she prefers. Practitioners who do not wish to provide contraceptive services are obliged to refer patients to other doctors who are willing to provide these services (GMC 1998).

What if the person seeking contraception is very young, as in Case 7.1? There are a number of ethical issues to consider here. What is in Lucy's best interests? One response might be that she is too young to be sexually active: she is not old enough to understand the nature and consequences of sex; she will regret her actions later; she is at increased risk of pregnancy and sexually transmitted diseases; and that it is surely not in her best interests to do anything which will facilitate her becoming sexually active. There may be concerns about the voluntariness of her decision to have sex with her boyfriend—he may be coercing her, or she may be swayed by popular images emphasizing young women's sexuality. If she does not wish her parents to know of her activities, she will have to deceive them, which may weaken trust within the family relationships.

On the other hand, Lucy may be very mature. She may have been in a relationship with her boyfriend for some time and the decision to have intercourse may be one that she has deliberated about. The fact that she has come for contraceptive advice prior to having intercourse suggests that this is a well-considered decision. In this case, it may not be in Lucy's interests to withhold contraceptive advice or to give her a lecture about the rights and wrongs of early intercourse.

One important factor to consider in this scenario is that of competence: is Lucy competent to make decisions about contraception? As discussed in Chapter 6, assessing a person's competence involves asking whether that person can:

(a) Understand the nature, purpose, and possible effects of the proposed treatment?

(b) Comprehend and retain information about the treatment?

(c) Believe what he or she is told and balance this information with other considerations (Mason and McCall Smith 1999)?

This assessment of competence is for adults; the standard for children, called Gillick competence, is very similar. If a GP is satisfied that the person they are treating, irrespective of their age, can fully understand the nature and implications of the proposed treatment, then that person is competent to make their own decisions without the permission or knowledge of anyone else, even the parents in the case of children.

Although the ruling was about giving consent for contraceptive services, the ruling covers all treatment for children under the age of 16; that is, Gillick-competent children under 16 years of age have the right to consent to any medical treatment. It is up to the treating doctor to decide whether or not a child is Gillick competent in relation to a specific treatment, based upon an assessment of the child's understanding of the nature of the proposed treatment and its implications, and the likely consequences if no treatment is given. One significant implication to discuss if a child does not wish her parents to know about a consultation is the potential effects of withholding information from or deceiving her parents.

Box 7.1 Gillick competence

The law recognizes that children mature at differing rates, and while some children may not be mature enough to make competent decisions about their medical care until they are well over the age of 16, others are capable of making those decisions at a younger age. Once a child is mature enough to make competent decisions, the parents no longer have the right to make decisions for the child, or necessarily to be informed about any medical care the child might have unless he or she agrees. This level of maturity is known as Gillick competence, after the ruling in the House of Lord in the case Gillick vs West Norfolk and Wisbech Area Health Authority. Mrs Gillick mounted a legal challenge to a Department of Health circular which said that in limited circumstances, doctors could give contraceptive advice to children under the age of 16 without parental consent. The trial judge ruled against Mrs Gillick, saying that a sufficiently mature child who understood the implications could give consent to receive contraceptive services. This verdict was overruled in the Court of Appeal, and then reinstated on further appeal to the House of Lords.

In the ruling, Lord Scarman stated that the parental right to determine whether or not their minor child below the age of 16 will have medical treatment 'terminates if and when the child achieves a sufficient understanding and intelligence to enable him or her to understand fully what is proposed' (in *Gillick vs West Norfolk and Wisbech Area Health Authority*, cited in Mason and McCall Smith 1999, p. 252).

Part of the importance of the Gillick ruling is the assurance of confidentiality that it brings; a child who is making his or her own decisions about medical care is entitled to receive the same high standard of confidentiality as anyone else. It may be important to emphasize the confidential nature of consultations in situations like those with Lucy; a teenager may be suspicious of adults in general unless specifically reassured that the entire consultation will remain private. Of course, in an ideal world children would be able to discuss important issues like sexuality with their parents, but whether or not this is possible, confidentiality must be assured.

Case 7.2

Mrs Shettleston comes to see her GP, Dr Grainger, about her daughter Maeve. Maeve is 15 years old and suffers from severe mental retardation and epilepsy. She has been menstruating for two years; her periods are heavy and irregular and at times seem to distress Maeve. Recently Maeve has started masturbating, and yesterday Mrs Shettleston found Maeve masturbating in the front garden watched by two teenage boys. Mrs Shettleston would like Dr Grainger to refer Maeve to a paediatric gynaecologist for a hysterectomy, to prevent any possible pregnancy and to avoid the problems associated with menstruation. She says that unless Maeve is sterilized, she will have to live in an institution as Mrs Shettleston cannot cope with the possibility of Maeve becoming sexually active.

The non-voluntary sterilization of people with mental disabilities raises a host of ethical issues. While GPs will not usually be involved in the final decision, they are often the first to be involved when a request like this is made. What kind of considerations are important here? The first is to recognize the potential for discrimination against people with mental disabilities. In general we are on hazardous moral ground when we make broad judgements about the fitness of different kinds of people to be parents. (See also below, on referrals for IVF.) Decisions about the care of people with mental disabilities are grounded in the interests of that person, so that decisions must be directed towards their good. This means that decisions about sterilization should be made on a case-by-case basis, and not rely solely on the fact of having a mental disability. It is important to try and find out whether menstruation is a significant medical problem for Maeve, in terms of menorrhagia or dysmenorrhoea, and what kind of medical solutions short of hysterectomy, are possible. If Maeve's menstruation is more of a problem for Mrs Shettleston in terms of inconvenience or distress, there is the risk of using serious and irreversible medical means to solve what is essentially a social problem.

In general, the least intrusive and most reversible kind of treatment, both for unwanted fertility and menstruation, should be tried.

Mrs Shettleston may be unprepared for Maeve's emerging sexuality, so that discussions and advice from those with experience in looking after people similar to Maeve may help her to cope with the situation in a less drastic way. Maeve's best interests are the most important consideration and must remain at the heart of any discussion about her medical care.

Abortion

Should the right to control fertility extend to abortion? Abortion has been legal in the UK since the 1967 Abortion Act (subsequently amended by the 1990 Human Fertilization and Embryology Act), so long as certain criteria are met.

The reasoning behind the abortion act is consequentialist; abortions can be justified in order to avoid serious harms (greater than the

---

Box 7.2 Situations in which abortion is legal in the UK

1 Continuation of the pregnancy would involve greater risks of injury to the physical or mental health of the woman or of any existing children of her family, than if the pregnancy were terminated.

2 There is a risk of grave permanent injury to the physical or mental health of the woman.

3 Continuation of the pregnancy would involve risk to the life of the woman greater than if the pregnancy were terminated.

4 There is a substantial risk that, if the child were to be born, it would suffer from such physical or mental abnormalities as to be severely handicapped.

The first condition requires the opinions of two registered medical practitioners and is valid until 24 weeks of gestation. The other conditions do not have any gestation restrictions. Conditions 2 and 3 require only one medical opinion.

harms of termination) that might follow if the pregnancy continues to full term. This way of looking at abortion recognizes that abortion is a significant moral act, but that it may be outweighed by other serious considerations. The gestational restrictions on condition 1 capture the discomfort that many people feel about late terminations for anything other than grave threats to the health of mother or child. The Act does not engage with two issues which lie at the heart of abortion debates: the status of the foetus, and the right of women to self-determination.

The central anti-abortion (pro-life) argument is that it is wrong to kill innocent human beings, and as foetuses are innocent human beings, it is wrong to kill foetuses (Marquis 1989). This rules out all abortions, no matter what the circumstances, and equates abortion with murder. Critics of this view argue that we should make a distinction between being a genetic human being and being a person. Human beings as persons have certain capabilities such as consciousness, the ability to communicate and reason, the capacity for self-directed activity, and the presence of self-awareness, and it is the presence of these capacities that confers moral status and guides our behaviour towards them (Warren 1999). Genetic human beings that lack these capacities (for example anencephalic babies) are not persons in this sense, and, it is argued, are not owed the same degree of moral consideration. If we accept that foetuses are potential rather than actual persons, they are owed some moral consideration, but not to the extent of overriding the interests of actual persons, such as pregnant women.

For some feminists, the status of the foetus is irrelevant to the abortion debate as it is the question of women's rights to self-determination which is the crucial issue. Even if we accept that a foetus is a person and has a right to life, this should not mean that women are obliged to remain pregnant:

> Having a right to life does not guarantee having either a right to be given the use of, or a right to be allowed continued use of, another person's body, even if one needs it for life itself.

> (Thomson 1971)

Without the freedom to end unwanted pregnancies, women may damage their health, be unable to care for existing children, and have their opportunities in life significantly reduced. For women who suffer failures of contraception or who are forced to have sex, abortion offers the only way to prevent these harms (Warren 2001).

No matter what the beliefs of individual practitioners, all women in the UK have the legal right to abortions. GPs are well placed to assist women in assessing the risks of abortion or of continuing with the pregnancy. GPs whose beliefs prevent them from referring women for abortions are obliged to disclose this to patients and to offer to refer them elsewhere (GMC 1998). The fathers of foetuses do not have any legal rights either to enforce or prevent the termination of that pregnancy. This position recognizes the importance of personal autonomy and the unacceptability of one person forcing another person to have or not have medical treatment.

Reproductive technologies

New technologies raise new ethical dilemmas, and reproductive technologies are no exception. Is infertility a natural misfortune or a treatable medical condition? Does our culture put undue pressure on both men and women to become parents to genetically related, disability-free children? Does treatment with reproductive technologies make the best use of limited medical resources?

There are many places where the boundary between medical and social problems is blurred, however infertility is a particularly emotive issue. Becoming a parent is central to many people's social identity and overall life plans, so that when this does not happen in a normal and natural way, the anxiety and grief can be overwhelming. The treatments for infertility are highly technical, involving a range of invasive interventions, and raising questions about acceptable genetic practices. There are few low-tech options, apart from donor insemination with informally acquired semen.

Adopting a medical approach to infertility commits women to reproductive technologies that may be harmful to their health, such as the hormonal manipulation necessary for egg harvesting and the increased risks of ectopic pregnancies and multiple births. As well as these physical harms, the nature of infertility treatments can be very alienating, reducing women to the status of producers of ova and incubators of embryos. There is a danger of exploiting the vulnerability that accompanies the desire to become pregnant. Most IVF centres have low success rates; less than one-quarter of treatments started result in a live birth (HFEA 2002). Given these statistics, it may be that patients' interests are better served by seeking alternative solutions, such as acceptance of biological childlessness or adoption, rather than submitting to infertility treatment. However, there may be considerable pressures upon couples to follow the treatment route given the premium our society places upon having a genetically related child of one's own.

These problems are magnified when we consider the wider implications of reproductive technologies. The existence of a medical solution (albeit fairly unsuccessful) creates its own demand: once a technology is available for those who are desperate to have children, people are at least implicitly encouraged to be desperate, to get access to the technology. The focus on producing individual children reinforces current social arrangements in which people have little access to meaningful relationships with children unless they become parents, and diverts attention away from the plight of other unrelated children (Sherwin 1992).

On the other hand, many people feel that having children is a fundamental part of human life, and that it is wrong to deny people the chance to try for a family. Having a child is sometimes referred to as a right. On this view, reproductive technologies are morally neutral instruments necessary for people to realize profoundly important human goals.

As well as providing infertile couples with the opportunity to have children, using reproductive technologies may avoid harms such as some genetic diseases, or allow parents greater choice about the children they have.

On a more practical level, GPs are involved in some aspects of infertility care once patients have made the decision to proceed. GPs are asked to provide information to fertility clinics (with consent from their patients) that might be relevant to the welfare of any child born as a result of the treatment.

Box 7.3 The right to found a family

Article 12 of the 1998 Human Rights Act states that: *'Men and women of marriageable age have the right to marry and to found a family, according to the national laws governing the exercise of this right'.*

The right to have children or the 'right to found a family' are often cited as reasons to justify the full range of infertility treatments. However, it is difficult to understand how a right to reproduce might work, in terms of whose duty it might be to ensure that pregnancy occurs. In the normal course of events a woman can only become pregnant with the co-operation of a man, but there is no general obligation upon men to make women pregnant. There is no way of guaranteeing the right to reproduce, as even with the best infertility clinics, successful outcomes are not assured. It is not clear whether this right implies that the state has an obligation to provide infertility services, and if so, to what level and with what restrictions, if any.

A more practical way of understanding this right is to think of it as a right of non-interference: no one has the right to prevent men and women of marriageable age from marrying and *attempting* to found a family.

Case 7.3

Mr and Mrs Barnett have been trying to achieve a pregnancy for 18 months, without success. Routine investigations to date have not identified any specific abnormalities in either partner, and they report frequent and satisfying sexual intercourse. They now wish to discuss the possibility of referral for further investigation and treatment at the local fertility centre.

After initial assessment at the fertility centre, Dr Jones receives a request for any information which may be relevant in helping the fertility centre to fulfil their obligations in relation to 'the welfare of any child who may be born as a result of the treatment (including the need of that child for a father), and of any other child who may be affected by the birth' (HFE Act 1990, Section 13, 5).

Case 7.3 (Cont.)

The leaflet goes on to explain that Dr Jones is not being asked to speculate on lifestyles or to assess her patients' suitability as parents, but merely to provide factual information, medical or otherwise, that might be relevant to the welfare of any child. The request is accompanied by a consent form signed by both Mr and Mrs Barnett.

Dr Jones knows that Mrs Barnett worked as a prostitute several years ago, and that her partner is aware of this. Dr Jones also knows that Mr Barnett has a child from a previous relationship and that he does not seem to have any contact with this child.

What should Dr Jones say in response to the request for information about the Barnetts? The final decision about whether to offer treatment is in the hands of the treating clinicians, however information provided by the GP, especially if questioning the welfare of any resulting child, may be very influential. In this situation, it is important that Dr Jones consciously avoids any prejudices she might have, for example about what kind of people make good mothers, or the responsibilities of fathers to their children from previous relationships. The GP's role is to consider if there is anything in either partner's history which might be a *significant* threat to the welfare of any child born as a result of this treatment.

The HF&E Act does not prohibit any category of patient from receiving treatment, that is there are no specific exclusions for age, sexual preference, patients without partners, or HIV positive patients. However, the HF&E Act does emphasize the need of children for fathers, which may exclude women who do not fit into traditional family patterns (Purdy 2001). Whether patients will receive funding through the NHS is a matter for local health authorities, which sometimes restrict funding to women below a certain age. The National Institute for Clinical Excellence (NICE) is developing a guideline on assessment and treatment for people with fertility problems, based upon evidence of clinical and cost effectiveness. The second draft of this guideline, released for public consultation in August 2003, recommends that couples meeting specific criteria (including maternal age restrictions) should be offered up to three complete cycles of NHS-funded IVF (NICE 2003). The final guideline is due for release in early 2004.

In pregnancy

Despite widespread beliefs that pregnancy and childbirth are not illnesses, in western societies the majority of pregnancies receive ever more sophisticated medical antenatal care, and the rate of interventions in childbirth continues to rise. GPs may have little influence once patients are admitted to secondary or tertiary care, but they are often the ones called upon to explain test results or advise on options offered by the hospital. This section looks at some of ethical issues which may be raised by antenatal care.

Antenatal screening in the form of blood tests and ultrasound examinations are a well-established part of antenatal care. However, as the range of tests has widened, a number of ethical problems have become apparent. Some antenatal screening is to detect disease in the mother, such as diabetes, anaemia, or various infections. These tests are relatively straightforward, as there are effective and largely acceptable treatments for most of the conditions detected. The ethics of anonymous HIV screening in pregnancy raises separate ethical issues that other authors have addressed (de Zulueta 2000). Other forms of screening are to detect abnormalities in the foetus (Aksoy 2001).

The reasoning behind the detection of foetal abnormalities is threefold:

(a) To inform prospective parents and help them to prepare for the birth of an affected child.

(b) To instigate treatment, either *in utero* or immediately after birth in a suitable centre.

(c) To allow termination of an affected foetus (Holt 1996).

In theory, screening provides information so that prospective parents can make informed choices between various options. In reality, very few detected abnormalities are suitable for *in utero* treatment, and the choice is between continuing with the pregnancy and having an affected child, or abortion. Current information indicates that the majority of women with pregnancies affected by disorders such as trisomy 13, 18, or 21, Tay-Sachs, anencephaly, spina bifida, thalassaemia, sickle cell anaemia, and sex chromosome abnormality terminate their pregnancies (Wertz and Fletcher 1998). It is not clear where the public

bility activists make the point that much of their disability is due
he way that society responds to disability, such as the lack of
ployment opportunities, barriers in the physical environment, and
scrimination. These social limits are far greater than those imposed
y their physiological disabilities.

However, it is not clear that quality of life judgements are the only reasoning that prospective parents use. As well as the welfare of the affected potential child, parents also consider whether or not they will be able
to cope with a disabled child in the family, and make comparisons
between having this affected child or trying for another pregnancy and
an unaffected future child (Gillam 1999).

There are concerns that antenatal screening and selective termination
are the beginnings of a slippery slope, and that once the door is opened
to foetal selection, the quest for perfect children will lead to termination
of foetuses with for example, lower intelligence or the wrong colour eyes.
At the moment, termination is offered for conditions which might cause
a severe handicap, but it can be impossible to predict the degree of
handicap, especially for conditions like spina bifida or Down's syndrome. More importantly perhaps, the consequences of the handicap
depend very much upon the social context. With advances in genetics, it
is likely that the range of conditions for which screening is offered will
increase; we will need informed and extensive public debate to develop
ethically responsible ways of responding to this development.

A second set of ethical issues are to do with the process of screening
and the benefits and harms to women.

Case 7.4

Mrs Nasser had her first pregnancy confirmed at 9 weeks and was booked at the
local hospital for shared care and a GP delivery. At 12 weeks she had a dating ultra
sound scan. At 16 weeks, she had blood taken for a number of tests. She was told
that there is a risk that her baby has Down's syndrome and that she should have
more tests. Mrs Nasser comes to see her GP, Dr Chu, concerned about what the
test results mean and that she may be advised to have an abortion.

The Midwives Information and Resource Service (MIDIRS) and the
NHS Centre for Reviews and Dissemination publish a range of leaflets
about informed choices in pregnancy and childbirth, emphasizing

would draw the line at the kind of abnorm.
consider termination. Some research sugg,
sumerism, with acceptance of selective term.
such as obesity, short stature, missing two finge.
talent (Henn 2000).

The first set of ethical issues raised by antenatal sc.
with questions about the kinds of lives that are consider.
and the implications of offering termination for affected,
framing the issue as one of choice, there is already an assun.
at least some people would choose not to have an affected foe.
is this assumption that raises concerns about eugenics and disc.
tion against the disabled. Eugenics is to do with improving the s̨
or the gene pool, either by controlling who reproduces, or by enco
aging or discouraging the reproduction of certain characteristics. Do.
screening for and offering terminations for conditions such as Down's
syndrome and spina bifida imply a eugenic policy trying to eliminate
these conditions from the population? The accepted view of genetic
counselling is that this should be non-directive and aimed towards
facilitating the uncoerced choice of the individuals concerned, rather
than trying to influence the overall make-up of the population.
However, there have been challenges to this view. First, non-directive
counselling is almost impossible in these situations, especially when the
only 'therapy' on offer is termination. The choices that parents face may
be limited by the foreseeable level of resources and support available to
assist them in raising a disabled child; where these are very low, the
decision to terminate may be driven by economic considerations. In
addition, outcome measures used to assess the effectiveness of genetic
counselling include measuring the incidence of genetic diseases.
A decreased incidence in affected live births is taken to be evidence of
successful counselling (Chadwick 2001).

What about the concern that antenatal screening and selective termination discriminate against disabled people? The argument here is
that if a foetus is aborted on the grounds that it would be better not
to be born at all than born with the disability, this implies that people
living with similar disabilities also have lives that are not worth living.
This is an implication which many people find offensive as it makes
a judgement about the value and quality of life of disabled people.

the importance of women receiving information and making well-informed decisions about all aspects of their care, including screening (MIDIRS 2002). Despite these efforts, there is not always time to fully explain what health professionals take to be routine tests, and it is only when a test is positive that the woman is suddenly faced with the full implications of having been tested. Mrs Nasser may not have been aware that she had had a test for Down's syndrome, or what a positive result means. The cut-off points for risk estimates vary between different screening services (in most areas the cut-off is 1/250), and different laboratories have different rates of false positives and false negatives. Even with a positive result, the chance of having an affected baby is approximately 1 in 60. Mrs Nasser may choose to decline further investigation, perhaps because she does not want to know whether or not she has an affected foetus, or because termination would not be an acceptable alternative. If she goes ahead with diagnostic testing, she faces the 1% risk of spontaneous abortion associated with amniocentesis.

Screening is usually assumed to be beneficial, in terms of detecting disease or disease precursor states and offering the chance for therapy. But as discussed, antenatal screening is a special case as at present there is little effective treatment for the majority of disorders that are diagnosed. (See also Chapter 4 for a discussion of the ethics of preventive care.)

The main reason that women have screening is for reassurance that their baby is healthy (MIDIRS 2002). When screening is negative, and the foetus given a clean bill of health, this can be immensely reassuring, but this degree of relief is unjustified as many abnormalities present at birth are not detected by routine antenatal tests, including one-third of pregnancies affected by Down's (MIDIRS 2002). Explaining these complexities together with the hazards and limitations of screening can be difficult and time-consuming, but it is important that women fully understand the implications of tests that they have. (See Chapter 6 for discussion of the importance of informed consent.)

Apart from issues to do with screening, pregnancy also raises issues to do with the dual interests of mother and foetus. Most pregnant women wish for the best possible outcome for their pregnancy and are prepared to comply with medical advice about lifestyle, diet, sporting activities, alcohol intake, and so on. Conflicts between the interests of the mother and those of the foetus are rare, but when they do occur, can be very challenging to deal with.

Case 7.5

Gemma is an 18-year-old patient who is a known intravenous drug user. She presents to the surgery with a 3 month history of amenorrhoea, and testing confirms pregnancy. Gemma wishes to continue with the pregnancy and expresses the hope that being pregnant will help her to break her habit and make a new start. Dr Grainger takes Gemma on as a shared care patient, but after the first hospital appointment, the consultant says that Gemma is a high risk patient and must receive all of her care from specialist services. Gemma makes no contact with either GP or hospital for several weeks. When she comes to see Dr Grainger, she says that she has been using drugs again, and that she does not want to attend the hospital clinic where she feels ostracized and despised.

Dr Grainger knows that Gemma's social supports are insecure and that there is a high risk of her continuing to use drugs.

Looking after patients with addictions poses many problems; these are magnified in pregnancy when maternal drug addiction or alcoholism can damage the foetus. Acting in the best interests of the foetus might suggest coercing Gemma into hospital admission or an invasive programme of monitoring to see whether she is complying with advice to remain drug free. However, there are two reasons why this approach is wrong. First, it is never right to force a woman to have treatment for the sake of her unborn child. We do not force parents or any other relatives to undertake medical procedures for the sake of their children or anyone else (for example to donate kidneys or marrow), therefore it does not seem right to demand that pregnant women place the interests of their foetus above their own interests. Of course, in many senses the interests of both mother and foetus would be served by ceasing drug use, but this does not justify coercing Gemma into treatment. Women have the right to accept or refuse any medical treatments, regardless of foetal outcome (Steinbock 2001).

The second reason why a coercive approach is wrong is consequentialist; offering support is far more likely to maintain a relationship with Gemma and lead to a better outcome than adopting a punitive attitude (Tong 1999).

Labour and delivery

Ethical issues may arise in relation to labour and delivery. Again, the majority of women accept medical direction about the most appropriate place of delivery, making their choices within the options on offer. Problems may arise when a woman wishes to deliver in a place or by a means that is not considered medically optimal. GPs are less likely to be involved in requests for elective Caesarean sections than requests for home deliveries, although both raise questions about how to respond to difficult or inappropriate requests. (See also Chapter 5 on inappropriate requests for treatment.) There is a significant difference between asking for a treatment, and refusing one. No patient has the right to demand a treatment on the NHS that his or her doctors do not feel to be indicated; there is no obligation upon obstetricians to perform Caesarean sections because the patient prefers this method of delivery. On the other hand, patients do have the right to refuse treatment, such as a Caesarean section, or delivery in a hospital, even if this is against medical advice and puts the foetus or mother or both in serious danger. Despite the general right to refuse treatment, there is a legal obligation to have a doctor or midwife present at all births, including home births.

What are the GP's obligations if a patient wishes to deliver at home against medical advice? First, the GP, or more likely the midwife, will usually have been aware of the woman's preferences throughout the pregnancy, in the context of an ongoing relationship. This provides opportunities for exploring the reasoning behind the decision and for ensuring that the woman fully understands the implications of her decision, in terms of possible harms or delayed access to tertiary care should this prove necessary. It is unlikely that a woman would make an arbitrary decision to knowingly increase the risks for herself and her baby without good reason, and it is part of her carer's duties to understand her reasons. Similarly, it is quite reasonable for the GP to act as medical advocate for the woman and her baby, explaining any risks openly and honestly (and remembering that we tend to overestimate risks). The aim should be to maintain trust whilst trying to reach an acceptable solution. Threatening withdrawal of services would not be acceptable, unless this was in the context of transferring care to a GP willing to support the patient in a home delivery.

If all attempts at negotiation fail, the GP still has a moral obligation to care for the patient. GP support will lead to the best possible outcome in the circumstances, even if those circumstances are not what the GP recommended. It would be wrong to abandon the patient because she has refused medical advice; just as patients who refuse advice in other circumstances (smokers with recurrent chest infections for example) are not abandoned. Although the baby-to-be-born does not have a legal claim upon the GP's services, the GP, having provided antenatal care, already has a stake in the baby's welfare. Attending the delivery will protect the baby's welfare more than staying away. As well as the moral obligation, there is a legal (terms of service) obligation on GPs to offer emergency care to anyone on their list, including women who have arranged for a home birth with a midwife, or another GP, or against advice.

Conclusion

In this chapter we have discussed a range of issues that arise in the fertility care of women and potential parents. Many of the final decisions are beyond the responsibility or control of GPs, but GPs are often well placed to understand their patients and their requests, and to act as advocates for them. In most practices, midwives are the primary carers for pregnant women, and they are often the ones who have to deal with issues as they arise. However, GPs play a vital role in looking after women's health related to fertility. We hope that the examples and discussion in this chapter will help to clarify some of the relevant considerations.

References

Aksoy, S. (2001). Antenatal screening and its possible meaning from unborn baby's perspective. *BMC Medical Ethics* 2(3). *http://www.biomedcentral.com/1472–6939/2/3*

Chadwick, R. (2001). Feminism and eugenics. Paper presented at the Beijing symposium on Feminist Approaches to Bioethics, Beijing November 2001.

General Medical Council. (1998). *Good medical practice.* General Medical Council, London.

Gillam, L. (1999). Prenatal diagnosis and discrimination against the disabled. *Journal of Medical Ethics* 25, 163–71.

Henn, W. (2000). Consumerism in prenatal diagnosis: a challenge for ethical guidelines. *Journal of Medical Ethics* 26, 444–6.

Holt, J. (1996). Screening and the perfect baby. In Frith, L. (ed.) *Ethics and midwifery: issues in contemporary practice*, pp. 140–55. Butterworth–Heinemann, Oxford.

Human Fertilisation and Embryology Authority. (2002). *Annual Report 2002. http://www.hfea.gov.uk/Downloads/default.htm*

Marquis, D. (1986). Why abortion is immoral. *Journal of Philosophy* **86**, 183–202.

Mason, J. and McCall Smith, R. (1999). *Law and medical ethics*, (5th edn). Butterworths, London.

MIDIRS. (2002). *Antenatal screening for congenital abnormalities: helping women to choose; Looking for Down's syndrome and spina bifida in pregnancy; and ultrasound scans—should you have one?* Midwives Information and Resource Service. *http://www.midirs.org/nelh/nelh.nsf/TOPICVIEWALL2C?OpenForm*

National Institute for Clinical Excellence. (2003). *Fertility: assessment and treatment for people with fertility problems* (Draft guideline) *http://www.nice.org.uk/cat.asp?c = 20092*

Purdy, L. (2001). Assisted reproduction. In Kuhse, H. and Singer, P. (ed.) *A companion to bioethics*. Blackwell Publishers, Oxford.

Sherwin, S. (1992). *No longer patient*, Temple University Press. Philadelphia, PA.

Steinbock, B. (2001). Mother–fetus conflict. In Kuhse, H. and Singer, P. (ed.) *A companion to bioethics*. Blackwell Publishers, Oxford.

Thomson, J. (1971). A defence of abortion. *Philosophy and Public Affairs* **1**, 47–66.

Tong, R. (1999). Just caring about maternal–fetal relations: the case of cocaine-using pregnant women. In Donchin, A. and Purdy, L.M. (ed.) *Embodying bioethics: recent feminist advances*. Rowman and Littlefield Publishers Inc, Maryland, MD.

Warren, M.A. (1999). On the moral and legal status of abortion. In Beauchamp, T. and Walters, L. (ed.) *Contemporary issues in bioethics*, (5th edn). Wadsworth Publishing Company, Belmont, CA.

Warren, M.A. (2001). Abortion. In Kuhse, H. and Singer, P. (ed.) *A companion to bioethics*. Blackwell Publishers, Oxford.

Wertz, D.C. and Fletcher, J.C. (1998). Ethical and social issues in prenatal sex selection: a survey of geneticists in 37 nations. *Social Science and Medicine* **46**, 255–73.

de Zulueta, P. (2000). The ethics of anonymised HIV testing of pregnant women: a reappraisal. *Journal of Medical Ethics* **26**, 25–6.

Further reading

Callahan, J. (1995). (ed.) *Reproduction, ethics and the law: feminist perspectives.* Indiana University Press, Bloomington, IN.

Dickenson, D. (2002). (ed.) *Ethical issues in maternal-fetal medicine.* Cambridge University Press, Cambridge.

Frith, L. and Draper, H. (2003). (ed.) *Ethics and midwifery: issues in contemporary practice,* (2nd edn). Butterworth-Heinemann Medical, Oxford.

Health Expectations (2001). **4**, 79–139. Special issue on participation in screening programmes and informed choice.

Journal of Medical Ethics (2001). **27**, ii2–ii36. *Supplement: the new ethics of abortion.* This series of articles explores various aspects of abortion including issues raised by disability screening and issues for service providers.

Williams, C. Alderson, P., and Farsides, B. (2002). Too many choices? Hospital and community staff reflect on the future of prenatal screening. *Social Science and Medicine* **55**, 743–53.

Chapter 8

Ethical issues at the end of life

Introduction

Case 8.1

Dr Jack Day has looked after Mr Glenn for many years and has an open and trusting relationship with him. Five years ago Mr Glenn was diagnosed with cancer of the prostate gland. Despite an initially positive response to therapy, he now has multiple bone secondaries. The oncologist treating him at the hospital has offered another course of radiotherapy, but Mr Glenn declined this, as the previous course made him feel very unwell, and he would rather not waste time having treatment which is not likely to make much of a difference to the length of his life. Mr Glenn lives with his wife who is well, but who finds it difficult to provide the assistance with dressing and bathing which Mr Glenn now needs. Dr Day visits Mr Glenn who has a fever and has been vomiting. The probable diagnosis is a urinary tract infection, which will respond to antibiotic treatment. Mr Glenn does not want any more treatments which will make him feel worse or prolong what he believes is the dying process. After discussion about the pros and cons of antibiotic treatment on

---

Case 8.1 *(Cont.)*

this occasion, Mr Glenn agrees to have the antibiotics but asks Dr Day not to let him suffer during the rest of the course of his illness. Dr Day assures him that he will provide pain relief and that it will be possible to keep him comfortable. However, Mr Glenn says that he hates being dependent and that once he becomes too weak to feed himself, he would like to end it all and to die with a little dignity. He wants to know if Dr Day can give him an injection when he becomes this weak.

Looking after patients who are terminally ill can be a very rewarding experience in general practice. Dying at home close to friends and relatives and cared for by familiar nursing and medical staff is something that many of us would prefer compared with dying in hospital. Looking after dying patients allows GPs to use the full range of their clinical, communication, and ethical skills as they meet the changing needs of patients. In this scenario, Mr Glenn does not wish to have treatment that he finds burdensome or life-prolonging. Dr Day respects his wishes, tailoring his treatment to meet Mr Glenn's ends. For Mr Glenn, the request for an assisted death may seem a natural extension of the good care that he has received from Dr Day, but for Dr Day, the request raises ethical issues.

We know that requests for help in dying are relatively common in general practice. An English study found that 64% of GPs had received a request for help in hastening death at some stage during their careers (Ward and Tate 1994). In the Netherlands, where euthanasia was first protected from prosecution and later legalized, 97% of GPs had discussed euthanasia or assisted suicide with patients over the past five years, with 73% receiving explicit requests in that period (van der Wal *et al.* 1992). It is hard to know whether the difference between England and the Netherlands is solely due to the illegal status of euthanasia in England, or whether the legal situation in the Netherlands has allowed people to talk more openly about their wishes.

How do GPs respond to these requests? In the English study, 30% of the GPs who were asked to hasten death complied with this request (Ward and Tate 1994). As we might expect, figures are higher from the Netherlands, where 47% of GPs performed euthanasia or assisted suicide at least once in a five year period (van der Wal *et al.* 1992).

When GPs are asked about their support for euthanasia and assisted suicide, support for legalization ranges from 40% in Australia and 35% in the UK (Ward and Tate 1994) to 12% in Northern Ireland (McGlade *et al.* 2000). However, not all of those supporting the legalization of euthanasia and assisted suicide would themselves be willing to perform these acts.

This brief statistical summary highlights some of the ethical issues to do with dying. Many people fear dying and turn to doctors for help in shortening the process. Doctors are then faced with conflicting ethical imperatives. Respect for the patient's autonomy and compassion for their suffering suggest that the ethical response is to honour these requests. On the other hand, assisting a patient to die may undermine respect for human life and ignore injunctions against killing. In this chapter we examine the range of ethical responses to requests for assistance in dying and discuss some of the conflicting ethical values raised by such requests. In the second part of the chapter we look at theoretical frameworks for classifying end of life decisions and acts, and discuss some of the arguments for and against the legalization of euthanasia.

Ethical responses to requests for assistance in dying

We may be tempted to think that euthanasia should not be acknowledged as a legitimate medical request, and that it is a question of personal values whether or not you agree with euthanasia. Of course, the situation is far more complex than this. The decision to perform or not perform euthanasia is not a routine part of general practice, but responding to a request from a patient takes place within the same framework of values that inform all general practice.

First of all, the well-being of the patient must be considered. It is important to acknowledge the distress which has prompted the call for help, irrespective of the practitioner's views about the acceptability of euthanasia. This can be difficult as few people, GPs or otherwise, welcome discussions about dying. The GP may be the only person with whom the dying patient feels free to voice their distress. Patients may fear upsetting their relatives with open talk of death, or their carers may close off any conversations. Providing support at this time, and accepting the way that the patient feels, are significant responsibilities of the doctor–patient relationship. Voicing a request for assistance in dying takes courage on the part of the patient, and trust that the GP will at least listen and not turn away.

Encouraging patients to discuss their fears and concerns is the first step towards alleviating them. Fear of pain is an important issue, but may be less important than fear of futile or unbearable suffering, loss of dignity, being a burden to others, and loss of control or dependency (van der Wal *et al.* 1992; McGlade *et al.* 2000). Promoting the patient's well-being in this situation requires understanding their fears, and also understanding how the patient him- or herself views these fears in relation to their values: do dependency and loss of control provide the opportunity to receive care from others, or are they a sign of weakness? Once the fears are identified, it is possible to see which of these can be helped by medical care, and to identify treatable causes, such as excess pain or previously unidentified depression. An important part of dying well is coming to terms with one's life and making some sense of it all. Sometimes the distress of the dying is due to psycho-spiritual issues like this rather than physiological pain.

In terminal illness, it may be difficult to consider the importance of patient autonomy, yet loss of control can be one of the most distressing aspects of illness. Part of Mr Glenn's distress may stem from receiving intimate personal care from his wife, when the established pattern in their relationship has been for him to care for her. He may find personal care from a stranger more acceptable than this role reversal with his wife. There may be no control over the progression of the disease, but autonomy may be respected by offering patients participation in decisions about their care and treatment. Even if the patient does not wish to participate in decisions, keeping him or her fully informed about the process of care is an important way of showing respect.

What if, after acknowledging the distress, and investigating and trying to alleviate the causes, the patient persists in their request for medical assistance in dying (Bascom and Tolle 2000)? What kind of values might inform a GP's response to a request like this? Respect for autonomy requires that patients' competent and informed decisions about medical care should be accorded significant weight. Being autonomous means being able to make significant decisions about one's own life, according to the values that have informed that life. When the period of life remaining is very short, it is surely up to the person concerned to act according to their values, and to be the judge of whether or not the burdens of their life outweigh the benefits. However, there are limits to the interventions that patients may request. While patients have an absolute right to refuse treatment, even life-saving treatment, they do not have a right to be given specific treatments. There are many situations in which it may be justified to deny patients interventions that they have requested; for example when there is no evidence that the intervention is efficacious, when it is not medically indicated, or when providing the intervention violates the deeply held beliefs of the practitioner.

Belief in the wrongness of killing runs deep in our society. This is often referred to as the sanctity of life doctrine, implying theological roots, although it is not clear that there was a general prohibition against killing in the early Judaeo–Christian tradition (Stoffell 2001). What we do have from the religious traditions is a belief in the moral value of life, and the notion that life is a gift which humans do not have the right to destroy. Secular traditions place an equally high premium upon the value of human life. The duty not to kill is grounded in the value that we place upon human capacities, such as self-determination, and is recognized in rights theories by the right of individuals to personal liberty and freedom from interference. A utilitarian might argue that killing is wrong because overall the effect of killing upon a society will bring more harm than good. The value that we accord to human life is reinforced by the values of medicine, dating back at least to the Hippocratic injunction to do no harm. The goals of medicine are directed towards protecting and preserving life, rather than intentionally ending it.

Despite these beliefs about the prima facie wrongness of taking life, most societies do make some exceptions. Killing another person in self-defence, or killing opponents in a just war are examples of killing that we usually do not condemn. This suggests that taking life is not always wrong, but that we need to examine the circumstances with care, to think about the motives as well as the outcome of acts which result in a person's death. In terms of responding to a request to end a life, there may be a range of motives which come into play, some of which are morally justified. Compassion for the person suffering is the motive which sits most easily within the framework of medical values. Medical care in general aims to relieve suffering, and many people think that performing euthanasia can best be understood in the context of providing a release from unbearable suffering. Good palliative care can provide a comfortable death for many people, but there are those who have intolerable symptoms or uncontrolled pain. Withholding medical assistance in dying for these cases condemns the person to extra hours or days of misery, whereas a compassionate response might be to end the suffering. Given the current illegality of euthanasia in the UK, any compassionate acts to end life are supererogatory (above and beyond the call of duty) rather than obligatory. Doctors must relieve suffering to the best of their ability but they are not morally obliged to take on the moral burden of killing a person, or to jeopardize their livelihoods by illegal acts, even if motivated by compassion.

We have already mentioned the importance of respect for patient autonomy at the end of life. Respecting a person's considered and repeated request to die might be another morally defensible motive for euthanasia. Here the justification would lie in the importance of allowing people to be self-determining, and in helping them to reach their goals if they are unable to fulfil these without assistance. Euthanasia activists refer to this as the right to death with dignity, or the right to die. The claim is that as we value having control over other aspects of our lives, it is equally, if not more important, to also have control over the timing of our deaths. It is not clear how helpful the language of rights is in this context. A right to die (as in a right to euthanasia) is a positive right, implying that someone must have a corresponding duty to perform euthanasia. However, as discussed above, doctors do not have a duty to perform euthanasia, so it is difficult to see what practical meaning a right to die might have.

What are some of the implications if we accept a right to die? There would need to be a general duty on the medical profession to perform euthanasia as the correlative to the patient's right. This kind of legal duty might weaken the capacity of doctors to be moral actors. If the right to die relies solely upon a patient expressing a wish to die, the doctor's feelings as to whether or not euthanasia is an appropriate moral response in this case become irrelevant. Doctors become involved purely for their technical skills rather than as people with a moral stake in the decision. The doctor would have a duty to respect the wishes of the patient, irrespective of their own views about the person's suffering. In contrast, euthanasia motivated by compassion places some of the responsibility for the decision to act with the doctor, in conjunction with a request for euthanasia from the patient. However, giving doctors control over the decision is unacceptably paternalistic to those who believe that patients should have the responsibility for deciding to end their lives.

What is euthanasia?

In the previous section we used the term 'euthanasia' to refer to the intentional ending of patient's life by medical means, at their request and to avoid suffering, as for example would have occurred if Dr Day gave Mr Glenn a lethal injection. This is the way the term is commonly used; a more accurate description of Dr Day's act, should he perform it, would be voluntary active euthanasia. Voluntary euthanasia is distinguished from non-voluntary euthanasia.

Box 8.1 Classifications of euthanasia

Voluntary euthanasia

Acting on the request of a person to end their life, usually by administration of a lethal drug. The request is generally made in the context of unbearable pain or suffering and/or a terminal illness.

Non-voluntary euthanasia

Acting to end a person's life in the absence of invitation or consent to do so. The person dying is usually incompetent. The doctor or proxy decision-maker believes this is what the person would want and/or that death is in their best interests. The decision is generally made in the context of terminal illness, severe disability, or brain injury.

These two types of euthanasia are further classified into active or passive euthanasia. Active euthanasia refers to the intentional adminis-tration of a lethal substance, such as an injection of a muscle relaxant, potassium chloride, or a high dose of opioids. In active euthanasia, it is the action of the person administering the euthanasia which causes death, irrespective of the underlying disease process.

Passive euthanasia refers to shortening of life by an omission to act. This may include:

(a) Not treating a treatable illness, for example not treating Mr Glenn's infection, if he then died of septicaemia.

(b) Withdrawal of treatment, for example withdrawing food and fluids from a person in a persistent vegetative state.

(c) Refusals of treatment, for example a person with motor neurone disease refusing ventilation during a chest infection (Mason and McCall Smith 1999).

In passive euthanasia, the person's death is caused by the underlying disease rather than by a substance administered by another person.

Passive euthanasia is widely accepted in many countries including the UK, where 'allowing nature to take its course' is both legal and a usual part of medical practice. In contrast, active euthanasia is illegal and has variable acceptance. If the intent in both cases is to ensure the death of the patient, why do we view the two practices so differently?

The distinction between active and passive euthanasia relies on finding a moral difference between an act and an omission, along the lines that we are morally more responsible for the consequences of our actions than we are for consequences that occur if we fail to act. If a patient dies because a doctor gives them a lethal drug, the doctor has killed that person. If a patient dies because a doctor does not give a life-saving drug (or withdraws a life-sustaining treatment), then it is the disease rather than the doctor who has killed the patient. Action implies direct control, whereas with an omission, even though death may be predicted, death is not necessarily ensured by the omission (for example, a person with advanced motor neu-rone disease may, against expectations, survive a chest infection which has not been treated with antibiotics and live for a few more days or weeks).

This distinction has proved very appealing both to medicine and to the law:

> The English criminal law ... draws a sharp distinction between acts and omissions. If an act resulting in death is done without lawful excuse and with the intent to kill, it is murder. But an omission to act with the same result and with the same intent is in general no offence at all.
>
> Lord Mustill in *Airdale NHS Trust v Bland*, cited in Mason and McCall Smith 1999, p. 430

Despite the appeal of allocating responsibility according to act or omission, there are some problems with this way of reasoning. First of all, it may be difficult to decide whether something is an act or an omission. Withholding antibiotics is straightforward, there is inaction on the part of the doctor, an omission to prescribe. Withdrawing treatment is not so straightforward. Turning off a ventilator is classed as an omission (a failure to provide life support), but turning off the ventilator is actually an act, in our common sense understanding of the term 'act', as is removing a nasogastric tube or an intravenous line.

Turning off a ventilator is a well-accepted example of allowing a person to die, but our thinking may be challenged by the following example comparing two cases of turning off a ventilator. First, a woman with advanced motor neurone disease who is ventilator dependent with no prospect of recovery asks her doctor to switch off the ventilator. He does so and the woman dies. Under the classification of acts and omissions, the doctor did not kill the patient but allowed her to die. Now imagine the same woman, who has a greedy son, impatient for his inheritance. He comes into her hospital room and switches off the ventilator and the woman dies. When confronted with his act, he says that he did not kill her, but he allowed her to die. Most people would reject his view of events and say that he deliberately killed her: without his action, the woman would have remained alive (Brock 2001). The problem is however, that the son performed exactly the same physical action as the doctor, so if the son killed the woman, then surely the doctor also killed the woman?

This example helps us to see the moral importance of motive: both the doctor and the son switched off the ventilator with the same intention, for the woman to die, but they had different motives, one morally justifiable and the other self-interested. Despite the clarity of the law in differentiating acts from omissions, the moral world is not so clear. The acts and omissions distinction says nothing about motive and does not always provide a guide to the difference between morally acceptable or unacceptable end of life decisions.

A recent pair of cases in the UK highlighted the paradoxes that arise as a result of the legal acts and omissions distinction.

Box 8.2 Similar cases with different outcomes: Ms B and Diane Pretty

Ms B and Diane Pretty both suffered from irreversible neurological diseases. Ms B had bled into her spinal cord and become paralysed and ventilator dependent. Diane Pretty had motor neurone disease. Both women wanted assistance with dying. Ms B wished to have her ventilator turned off, which would result in her death. Diane Pretty wanted her husband to assist her to commit suicide as she was no longer capable of physically acting on her own behalf.

The staff looking after Ms B did not agree with her wish to have her ventilator turned off, despite a psychiatric assessment that Ms B was fully competent. Ms B challenged the staff legally, leading to a ruling by a senior family judge that the NHS trust had acted illegally in not respecting her request to have treatment withdrawn. Subsequently Ms B was transferred to the care of a different medical team, her treatment was withdrawn, and Ms B died.

Diane Pretty sought legal assurances that her husband would not be prosecuted for assisting with her death. She took her case to the UK High Court, the House of Lords, and the European Court of Human Rights. None of these courts found in her favour, and she died without assistance from her husband.

Many commentators felt that the moral issues in these cases were very similar: both women were suffering and both women sought assistance with dying (Boyd 2002). The difference between their cases was that one happened to be dependent upon a machine whereas the other was not. This difference seems to be arbitrary rather than moral: why should the exact nature of the illness dictate whether or not a person can be helped to die? If suffering and a repeated request for help are sufficient in one case, why are these same moral considerations inadequate to ensure help in a similar case?

The doctrine of double effect

The reasons we have for performing actions are important moral considerations. The doctrine of double effect is a way of trying to distinguish between the intended and the unintended effects of an action, recognizing that sometimes an act with a good effect (such as pain relief) may also have an unintended ill effect (such as death). The effects (both intended and unintended) of actions which meet the conditions of the doctrine are considered by some to be morally acceptable, even if the unintended effects would otherwise not be morally acceptable. There are four parts to the doctrine.

Box 8.3 The doctrine of double effect

1 The act itself must be morally permissible.
2 The ill effect, while foreseen, must be unintended.
3 The ill effect must not be disproportionate to the good effect.
4 The ill effect is not the means by which the good effect is achieved.

The doctrine of double effect is an argument to justify medical actions which, while intending to relieve suffering, may also hasten death. The classic example is that of administering morphine to a terminally ill person, with the aim of relieving suffering but in the knowledge that the accompanying respiratory depression will hasten death. This fulfils all of the criteria of the doctrine:

(a) The administration of morphine for pain relief is a morally permissible action.

(b) The morphine is intended to relieve pain rather than cause respiratory depression.

Table 8.1 Voluntary death and medical aid in dying

Classification	Example	Moral justifications	UK legal status
Suicide	Self-killing by means such as hanging, drug overdose, or carbon monoxide poisoning. No involvement of others.	Right of individuals to self-determination; may be prudent or courageous.	Legal under the 1961 Suicide Act.
Physician-assisted suicide	Provision of means for patient to kill themselves, such as a prescription for self-poisoning, or insertion of an iv line for a patient to inject lethal drugs. Requires involvement of doctor.	Right of individuals to self-determination; assisting patient to achieve self-determination; compassion for suffering of individual.	Illegal under Section 2 (1) of the 1961 Suicide Act.
Passive euthanasia I: Refusal of treatment by competent person	Refusal of antibiotics in advanced malignant disease, or advance directive refusing resuscitation. No direct involvement of others.	Right of individuals to self-determination; duty of doctors to respect wishes of competent patient.	Legal under common law.
Passive euthanasia II: Withdrawing or withholding life-sustaining treatment from incompetent patient	Turning off ventilator in person with massive stroke, or withholding nutrition from a severely brain damaged patient. May require involvement of others.	Avoidance of burdensome or futile treatment; relief of suffering; best interests of patient to cease treatment; fair use of medical resources.	Legal under common law.

Active voluntary euthanasia	Doctor administering lethal dose of drug with aim of causing immediate death, at patient's request.	Right of individuals to self-determination; assisting patient to achieve self-determination; compassion for suffering.	Illegal.
Active non-voluntary euthanasia (person usually incompetent)	Doctor administering lethal dose of drug in absence of any request, for example actively killing severely disabled neonate.	Avoidance of burdensome or futile treatment; relief of suffering; best interests of patient to cease treatment; fair use of medical resources.	Illegal.
Doctrine of double effect	Doctor administering drugs with aim of relieving suffering, knowing that side-effect may be to hasten death.	Compassion for suffering; death foreseen but unintended.	Legal under common law.

(c) The good of relieving pain outweighs the loss of life in a patient who is already dying.

(d) The good effect, of relieving pain, is achieved by the action of the morphine rather than by the person dying.

The doctrine rules out active euthanasia, as in euthanasia the act (administering a lethal substance) is impermissible, death is an intended rather than an unintended consequence, and the good effect (relief of suffering) is achieved by means of the ill effect (killing the patient).

Both the medical profession and the law are comfortable with the doctrine of double effect as a way of dealing with medical treatments which simultaneously help the patient but also shorten life. Appeals to double effect provide a way for doctors to answer requests for help in ending a patient's pain or suffering, without falling foul of the law.

In practice however, it can be difficult to maintain the distinction between intended and unintended effects, and even more difficult to take this as the difference between morally permissible and impermissible killing. It may not be possible to differentiate between the relief of suffering caused by the morphine and the relief caused by death, because the two are often closely linked. Is the doctrine just a way of framing the issue so that we feel (legally and medically) comfortable with this form of active euthanasia? The doctrine of double effect seems to allow euthanasia using certain drugs (such as morphine) but not using other drugs (such as potassium chloride), that may be more suitable.

Table 8.1 lists the different kinds of actions that can end lives, giving examples and possible moral justifications for the actions. The table shows that the legal status varies between actions, although the moral justifications may be identical.

Practical aspects

Our discussion so far has covered some of the theoretical aspects of euthanasia, trying to clarify the moral considerations that are raised when lives are intentionally ended. In practice, issues are seldom clear, and GPs may be faced with making difficult treatment decisions without the benefit of knowing the wishes or the values of the patients they look after.

Case 8.2

Dr Schroeder is doing a locum for a busy urban practice. One evening he is called to the local nursing home to see an 83-year-old woman called Mrs Murray. The nurse who calls Dr Schroeder is from an agency; she has worked at the home on previous occasions but she is not very familiar with the patients. Mrs Murray had a stroke 14 months ago which left her with a moderate hemiplegia. She is sometimes incontinent and requires help with feeding. Her only daughter lives in France. Tonight Mrs Murray has a high fever and cough. She does not respond to questions from Dr Schroeder but resists undressing. Dr Schroeder examines Mrs Murray and makes a provisional diagnosis of pneumonia. Without treatment it is likely that Mrs Murray will die of her chest infection. Dr Schroeder asks if Mrs Murray has an advance directive or if there have ever been any discussions about treatment decisions in this kind of situation. There is no advance directive, nothing written in Mrs Murray's case notes, and the nurse has no idea of Mrs Murray's wishes regarding treatment. Dr Schroeder phones Mrs Murray's daughter in France. There is no reply.

What should Dr Schroeder do? Mrs Murray is not able to say what she wants in this situation, nor is there any indication of what her wishes might be. If she is not treated with antibiotics, she is likely to die. Dr Schroeder's first thought is to act in Mrs Murray's best interests, but this is difficult without any idea about her views of her own interests. Would Mrs Murray see pneumonia as a welcome release from a lonely and disabled life, or would she wish to be treated? Faced with a patient who is unable to make her preferences known, Dr Schroeder considers his patient's medical interests, which would be served by prompt treatment. In reaching his decision, Dr Schroeder considers the benefits and burdens of the treatment: oral antibiotics are not invasive or particularly burdensome, and the benefits are likely to be resolution of the infection and return to Mrs Murray's previous state of health. In the absence of further relevant information from relatives or those who usually care for Mrs Murray, acting for her medical good is the morally required response. Withholding treatment in this case would be an example of passive non-voluntary euthanasia.

If the circumstances were different, if perhaps Mrs Murray had heart failure and a second stroke which meant that she was unable to swallow, the balance between the benefits and burdens would change.

Treatment would involve insertion of a nasogastric tube or an intravenous line, and there would be less likelihood of recovery to her previous state of health. In these circumstances initiating a limited trial of treatment or withholding treatment may be morally justified. Situations like these require a careful assessment as to whether or not the patient is in the process of dying, in which case doctors are not obliged to initiate or continue treatments which are burdensome and likely only to prolong the process with no benefits to the patient (GMC 2002).

Advance directives

What if Dr Schroeder had found an advance directive indicating that Mrs Murray would refuse treatment such as antibiotics for life-threatening illnesses?

Box 8.4 Advance directives

Advance directives or living wills are statements (verbal or written) expressing a person's wishes about future medical treatment in the event that the person becomes disabled in some way. They are a mechanism for respecting patient autonomy at a time when the person is no longer able to make and/or communicate their wishes. Usually advance directives are used to describe limits to interventions, such as advance refusal of ventilation or CPR, or of antibiotics or parenteral food and fluids, but they may also be used to indicate that a person would like to receive life-prolonging treatment.

The purpose of advance directives is to enable individuals to participate effectively in decision-making and to control their medical care, even at a time when they are functionally no longer able to participate. Advance directives can lift the burden of decision-making from relatives and health care professionals. There are some disadvantages of advance directives:

1 Difficulties with giving unambiguous instructions covering every possibility, so that it may be impossible to know whether or not the current clinical situation is covered by the instructions.

Box 8.4 Advance directives *(cont.)*

2 Concerns that the intervening illness has caused a shift in the person's identity and their views and wishes, so that the person who made the advance directive in some sense no longer exists. If this is the case, the instructions made by the person prior to illness may no longer be relevant to the disabled person.

Advance refusals of treatment, if made by competent, well-informed patients, and clearly applicable to the current situation, should be respected. Advance requests for treatment do not carry the same force; doctors are not obliged to provide specific treatments because a person has requested such treatments, especially if medical opinion is that the treatment is not indicated or is futile.

Apart from the disadvantages listed in the box, the usefulness of advance directives is limited by two further factors. To date, not many people in the UK (less than 20%) have made advance directives, indicating that they are not a widely accepted form of decision-making (Mason and McCall Smith 1999). Secondly, there can be practical problems in establishing whether or not a person has made a directive, and then finding it in time to be useful in the decisions at hand. If the advance directive is stored with other important documents in a safe place, it is unlikely to be available to the treating doctors. If the directive is several years old, there may be concern that the person might have changed their mind. Despite these drawbacks, general practice may be the logical place for people to discuss their wishes about treatment at the end of life, with some record of these being kept with the patient's notes. Discussions which take place with a familiar GP or practice nurse at a time when the patient is relatively well may be very helpful in informing decisions about future care. Patients' wishes could be reviewed over time, for example during annual health checks, to make sure that the written information keeps up with any changes in the patient's condition.

Legalizing euthanasia and assisted suicide

At the moment in the UK, active euthanasia and assisted suicide are illegal, although as Table 8.1 shows, the moral justifications for these practices may be identical to the moral justifications for similar but currently legal practices such as passive euthanasia. In this section we discuss the arguments for and against the legalization of active euthanasia and assisted suicide.

The arguments in favour of legalizing active euthanasia draw upon many of the points that we have already discussed such as:

(a) The right to self-determination and the obligations of doctors to respect autonomous decisions.

(b) The duty to relieve suffering even if the only way to achieve this may cause the death of the patient.

(c) The difficulty of distinguishing between intended, and foreseen but unintended consequences, as per the doctrine of double effect.

(d) Apparent inconsistencies in the way that the law currently differentiates between people who may be assisted to die on the basis of morally arbitrary distinctions such as the presence or absence of life-supporting interventions.

In addition to these points, those in favour of legalization argue that the slippery slope of widespread euthanasia in the wake of legalization has not occurred in the Netherlands. Legalizing euthanasia would allow society to recognize the limits of medicine and enable people to discuss their end of life wishes more openly and honestly. Finally, they point out that at times, passive euthanasia, such as withdrawing food and fluids, may condemn a dying person to an apparently more prolonged and unpleasant death than administering active euthanasia.

With regard to assisted suicide, the law and society currently accept that people have the right to kill themselves, and that this may be morally justifiable at times, but that it is not legal to assist a suicide. What about people such as Diane Pretty, who want to kill themselves but are not able to because of illness or disability? Does this imply that the current law against assisted suicide discriminates against people who are unable to kill themselves (Doyal and Doyal 2001)?

Those who oppose the legalization of active euthanasia respond to each of these points. We have discussed some of these arguments above, such as the general prohibitions against killing and the problem of framing the discussion in terms of a right to die. There are also a number of consequentialist arguments that refer to the probable harmful effects that might occur following legalization of euthanasia. The slippery slope argument revolves around the concern that once we remove the prohibition against all active killing, there is no logical place to draw a line between acceptable and unacceptable killing. The circumstances in which euthanasia was performed might then expand to include cases that most people would agree are not acceptable. For example, doctors would have no logical grounds for refusing euthanasia to any person who requested it, including those who are not terminally ill. People with chronic illnesses and mental illness would become potential candidates. The very fact that euthanasia was legal might act as a pressure to request euthanasia, especially if the resources to support and care for these people were limited. The other group potentially affected by the slippery slope are those who are not competent: once we accept active involuntary euthanasia for this group, there may be a temptation to shift from considerations of suffering and burdensome treatment to increasingly narrow quality of life judgements about the kinds of lives that are worth living.

The legalization of euthanasia might erode trust in doctors, especially amongst the aged and vulnerable, who might feel that any discussions about dying were covert invitations to accept euthanasia. There are also questions about the fallibility of medical diagnoses and the uncertainty of predictions about suffering, that make it difficult for people to make truly informed decisions. Finally there are concerns that performing euthanasia may have damaging moral and psychological effects upon doctors.

Both those in favour of and those against legalizing euthanasia appeal to evidence from the Netherlands to support their cases. It is intriguing that despite more than ten years of experience, opinion remains divided about the effects of making active euthanasia available. There does not seem to be any evidence that the slope is as slippery as feared, although there have been cases of euthanasia performed on people with mental rather than terminal illness, and there may be under-reporting of non-voluntary euthanasia.

Would legalizing assisted suicide avoid some of the pitfalls of active euthanasia? If people who wished to commit suicide could be assisted by another person, including but not limited to doctors, this would remove any necessary connection with the medical profession. For doctors, this might be more acceptable than being the ones nominated to assist with dying. On the other hand, there is evidence to suggest that the public in the UK would prefer euthanasia, rather than assisted suicide, to be available. This may reflect the reluctance on all sides to be involved in actively helping someone to die (Mason and McCall Smith 1999).

Assisted suicide leaves control over dying with the person concerned, so that there is less likelihood that they might have a last minute change of mind. What about the moral responsibility of those involved? If a GP writes a prescription for a lethal dose of drugs, in response to a request from a patient, is that GP as responsible as she would be performing active euthanasia? Certainly some forms of assisted suicide create a gap between the doctor's actions and the patient's death, leaving the patient as the final moral actor. But what if the patient is, for example, unable to swallow and needs an intravenous drug? In this case the doctor's actions are much closer to the death of the patient, and we can imagine scenarios where there is almost no difference between assisted suicide and active euthanasia.

Conclusion

Assisted dying raises many difficult ethical issues, complicated by various intersections with the law which leave some practices legal and others illegal. Active euthanasia undoubtedly occurs in the UK and elsewhere; whether the incidence of this would change with legalization is unknown. We believe that there can be morally justifiable forms of medically-assisted dying, but as these relate to the context and to the motives of the doctor concerned, it is very hard to develop a framework in which euthanasia 'for the right reasons' would be legal, whilst maintaining the prohibition against other forms of killing. Assisted suicide avoids some of the dilemmas for doctors, but has its own problems, not least of which would be responding to failed assisted suicides.

Irrespective of the legal situation, GPs have a major role to play in providing care to people at the ends of their lives. Compassionate and sensitive medical care can reduce much of the fears and suffering of the dying; over and above the provision of this care at present remains a private matter between GP and patient.

References

Bascom, P. and Tolle, S. (2000). Treatment at the end of life. In Sugarman, J. (ed.) *Ethics in primary care*. McGraw-Hill, New York, NY.

Boyd, K. (2002). The law, death and medical ethics. Mrs. Pretty. and Ms. B. *Journal of Medical Ethics* **28**, 211–12.

Brock, D. (2001). Medical decisions at the end of life. In Kuhse, H. and Singer, P. (ed.) *A companion to bioethics*, pp. 231–41. Blackwell Publishers, Oxford.

Doyal, L. and Doyal, L. (2001). Why active euthanasia and physician-assisted suicide should be legalised. *British Medical Journal* **323**, 1079–80.

General Medical Council. (2002). *Withholding and withdrawing life-prolonging treatments: good practice in decision-making*. General Medical Council, London. *http://www.gmc-uk.org/standards/default.htm*

Mason, J. and McCall Smith, R. (1999). *Law and medical ethics*, (5th edn). Butterworths, London.

McGlade, K., Slaney, L., Bunting, B., and Gallagher, A. (2000). Voluntary euthanasia in Northern Ireland: general practitioners' beliefs, experiences, and actions. *British Journal of General Practice* **50**, 794–7.

Stoffell, B. (2001). Voluntary euthanasia, suicide and physician assisted suicide. In Kuhse, H. and Singer, P. (ed.) *A companion to bioethics*, pp. 272–9. Blackwell Publishers, Oxford.

van der Wal, G., van Eijk, J., Leenen, H., and Spreeuwenberg, C. (1992). Euthanasia and assisted suicide 1. How often is it practised by family doctors in the Netherlands? *Family Practice* **9**, 130–4.

Ward, B. and Tate, P. (1994). Attitudes among NHS doctors to requests for euthanasia. *British Medical Journal* **308**, 1332–4.

Further reading

BMA publications on ethical issues at the end of life, including euthanasia, physician-assisted suicide and treatment withdrawal. Access these at *http://www.bma.org.uk/ap.nsf/Content/pas+project+-+publications*

Doyal, L. and Doyal, L. (2001). Why active euthanasia and physician assisted suicide should be legalised. *British Medical Journal* **323**, 1079–80.

General Medical Council (2002). *Withholding and withdrawing life-prolonging treatments: good practice in decision making.* General Medical Council, London. *http://www.gmc-uk.org/standards/default.htm*

Journal of Medical Ethics (2002). **28**, 232–43. Special clinical ethics symposium: the case of Ms B. Series of six articles discussing the request by Ms B for the withdrawal of life-sustaining treatment.

Keown, J. (1997). (ed.) *Euthanasia examined : ethical, clinical, and legal perspectives.* Cambridge University Press, Cambridge.

Chapter 9

Role conflicts in general practice

Introduction

Thus far we have focused principally on the ethical issues that arise out of GPs' relationships with patients. Yet many aspects of GPs' work are not undertaken directly with patients. For example, GPs take part in research projects, they attend continuing education events, they consult with patients' families, and they manage the financial and administrative sides of their practices. As they do these things, they develop and maintain relationships with a wide range of individuals and organizations. Such relationships create multiple, and sometimes conflicting, obligations. This chapter explores the ethical issues that can arise because of these multiple obligations.

We will consider these issues through the ethical lens provided by a discussion of conflicts of interest. The chapter reviews the concept of a conflict of interests and explores the ways in which such conflicts arise in five specific circumstances—contact with relatives, the GP and family responsibilities, relationships with colleagues, inducements to participate in research, and gifts from pharmaceutical companies.

Conflicts of interest in general practice

We have explored the ethical implications of the GP's role from a number of angles in this book. We have discussed the nature of the doctor–patient relationship and the centrality of trust in that relationship, the importance of confidentiality, the meaning of beneficence and respect for autonomy, and analysed how GPs can manage ethically the competing demands for their time and resources. In all of these discussions, the GP's primary role, and therefore her principal obligation, is the care of patients.

However, while a GP's primary responsibility may lie with patients, this is not his *only* responsibility. As noted above, work in general practice is diverse, involving interactions with a range of individuals and organizations that create a variety of obligations, responsibilities, and interests. In addition, most GPs have private and social lives outside their work and these aspects of their lives also generate obligations and expectations. The following list indicates the breadth of roles that GPs fill and the potential for conflict; we will return to these examples later in the chapter.

(a) Dr Jones wants to spend time with her young children.

(b) Dr Shah and Dr Schroeder are concerned about patient safety, but also about their own standing in the medical community.

(c) Dr Chu and his practice gain from their contact with a pharmaceutical company.

(d) Dr Grainger receives fees for enrolling patients in a clinical trial.

(e) Dr Carter wants to enjoy his holidays.

The fact that general practitioners are party to a variety of relationships and occupy a number of roles always has the potential to create tension and conflict. But, the *potential* for conflict need not always translate into *actual* conflict.

Box 9.1 Conflict of interests

A conflict of interests is a set of conditions in which professional judgement concerning a primary interest (such as a patient's welfare or the validity of research) tends to be unduly influenced by a secondary interest (such as financial gain).

(Thompson 1993)

Each component of this definition is important. First, Thompson distinguishes between primary and secondary interests. *Primary interests* are those which arise out of specific professional duties. The obvious primary interest that GPs have is the health of their patients. However, particularly when they are not directly providing patient care, GPs may have other professional duties that are related to different primary interests. For example, they may supervise students and GP registrars or they may undertake research. These roles generate different sets of obligations, for example, the obligation to educate students and junior doctors to a high standard, or the obligation to conduct rigorous research. Some GPs will serve on professional bodies, for example, disciplinary bodies, and these GPs will have obligations to uphold high standards for the profession. The precise content of these interests may be debatable and occasionally there will be conflict between these primary interests. Nonetheless, what such interests have in common is that they arise out of the GP's professional roles and they should be the principal consideration in any decision the GP makes.

Box 9.2 Professional interests in general practice

Primary interests for GPs

1 The health of patients.
2 The integrity of research.
3 The education of students.
4 High professional standards for general practice.

Secondary interests for GPs

1 Financial gains.
2 Prestige.
3 Public recognition.
4 Friendships.

Thompson also acknowledges that there are *secondary interests* that may influence the GP's judgement. He has in mind interests such as financial gain, personal prestige, public recognition, and friendship bonds. There is nothing morally suspect about these interests in and of themselves. For example, good professional practice can include the wish to be respected and valued by one's peers.

The third component of the definition, the *undue influence* that secondary interests may have on professional judgement, describes the conditions under which a conflict of interests arises. Secondary interests may play a legitimate role in our decisions. There is only a conflict of interests when decisions which ought to be for the most part influenced by primary interests, such as patients' welfare, come to be shaped mainly by secondary interests, such as financial gain.

Finally, Thompson says that a conflict of interests is a *set of conditions*. This focuses our attention on the circumstances in which conflicts arise, rather than on the actual behaviour of doctors (Kassirer and Angell 1993). GPs who may benefit financially from enrolling patients in a randomized control trial that imposes significant burdens on patients have a conflict of interest regardless of whether they actually do go ahead and enrol patients or not. As Kassirer and Angell suggest, it is: 'circumstances [that] determine whether there is a conflict of interest, not the outcome' (1993, p. 570).

In some respects, conflicts of interest are unlike other sorts of moral conflict, such as the following conflict between respecting a patient's choice to refuse care, and acting in the most beneficent manner toward that patient.

Case 9.1

Mrs Duke, a patient in her late sixties, is an infrequent attender at the Gordon Road Practice. One day she presented to Dr McDonald with abdominal distension and anorexia. On examination, Dr McDonald found a large mass and ascites. Dr McDonald thought that the most likely diagnosis was ovarian cancer. She explained this to Mrs Duke and advised that some investigations would help to confirm the diagnosis and then it would be possible to work out what, if any, treatment would be recommended. Mrs Duke refused to have any investigations or to see a specialist for further assessment. She eventually died several months later.

In this scenario, there are two competing priorities—respect for patient autonomy and beneficence. In principle, both are equally important, and the dilemma here is to decide on which principle to focus. Conflicts of interest, however, do not have this equality of priority. Usually, it is clear that one interest—for example, patient health—should take precedence, and the problem is how to ensure that other interests do not override the doctor's primary obligation to care for his patient.

One set of interests that we can add to Thompson's secondary list is non-financial self-interests. A GP's interest in her own welfare will not always relate to financial issues. It may be, for example, that the personal interests the doctor wishes to promote concern her quality of life (for example, how many sessions she works); her safety (to what extent she exposes herself to infections, or to home visits in potentially dangerous situations); or her emotional and psychological well-being (how much she takes to heart her patients' burdens). In each of these cases, the GP may be faced with the realization that her legitimate concern for her own well-being may not be in her patients' best interests.

These issues are important, not least because there has been increasing recognition in recent years that some GPs are inclined to pay too little attention to their own well-being. While once it may have been acceptable to work 80 hour weeks, never take recreation leave, ignore the needs and wishes of families, and devote oneself totally to medicine, today there is more emphasis on the need for doctors to practise self-care, by ensuring that they take adequate leave, work sensible hours, and develop interests outside of medicine. The moral justifications for self-care are complex. In part, doctors' interest in their own welfare can be justified by arguing that the GP who leads a balanced life provides better care for patients than the GP who is chronically overworked. This argument retains the health and care of patients as the primary interest. A second justification for self-care by doctors focuses on the rights that all people have to acceptable working conditions and adequate leisure. In daily life, such conceptual clarity is rare, and the line between self-interest in the interests of patients, and self-interest as an end in itself, is often blurred. Deciding how much to give to self and how much to patients will always be a difficult issue.

Why should we be concerned about conflicts of interest?

Conflicts of interest are significant ethically for a number of reasons. First, they can place at risk the relationship of trust between GP and patient. We have explored the concept of trust in detail in Chapter 2; here is sufficient to note that patients expect that doctors will have their best interests at heart. The fulfilment of that expectation is central to the maintenance of trust. If patients perceive their GP to have divided loyalties—whether or not the GP is actually influenced by secondary interests—they may question the faith they place in their GP and in the profession generally (Lemmens and Singer 1998).

Secondly, patients are in a relatively powerless position *vis a vis* their medical practitioners; apprehension, weakness and fear, coupled to the knowledge imbalance between doctor and patient, means that patients often need to trust that their doctor will act for them when they are unable to act for themselves (Pellegrino 1987, 1994). In these situations, patients may need to trust their GP's judgement more than they might, say, trust the opinion of the car mechanic who fixes their car. Again, the possibility that the GP will have interests other than their patients' interests can undermine the necessarily trusting relationship between doctor and patient.

Finally, in certain situations secondary interests can become so persuasive that we might almost expect some doctors to succumb to them. Financial inducements that, in normal circumstances, might not tempt a doctor, may become compelling if a doctor discovers that he has managed his personal finances poorly and over-committed himself by taking out a large mortgage on his new house. Understanding and recognizing potential conflicts of interest can help us to avoid them.

Some specific examples

In this section we provide examples of conflicts of interest. We follow this with a discussion of how to evaluate and resolve conflicts of interest. These examples clearly do not exhaust the range of conflicts GPs may encounter in their work. They are set out here to indicate the types of conflicts GPs routinely face and to provide material for the sections that follow.

Dealing with relatives

Providing care to families as well as individuals can lead to conflicts of interest. The care of elderly relatives provides one example; a woman caring for her 84-year-old mother who is mildly demented and who tends to wander at night might request a sedative, both to keep her mother safe in bed at night and also to allow the carer to have peaceful nights. There are several considerations which are important with this kind of request. First the GP has to determine the nature and extent of the problem. This can be difficult if the history is only available from the carer and it is possible that she is exaggerating in order to make sure her request is successful. The GP has to make an assessment about the trustworthiness of the carer, based on her previous knowledge of both her and her mother. It is also important to work out who is the patient in this context—is it the mother who may be in danger from wandering, or the daughter who is not getting enough sleep? A home visit may be necessary to assess the kinds of dangers that are present in the home. The request may be a cry for help from the carer, which she hopes will trigger a move towards residential care for her mother. Factors of this kind all feed into an ethical response, and as with other situations, there may be no ideal solution. Some kind of weighing up of the harms of sedatives versus the benefits of avoiding a nocturnal accident will be part of the decision, as will an assessment of the mother's understanding of the situation and willingness to take sleeping tablets.

Consultations with children can also trigger conflicts of interest, for example if the mother of an asthmatic child refuses to allow her child to use a steroid inhaler, because of a belief in the harmfulness of steroids. Doctors are obliged to act in the best interests of a child who is a patient, even if this goes against the wishes of the parents. In practice this can be difficult as, at least for young children, treatment is mediated through the parents. In situations where extreme harm may come to the child, the child can be made a ward of the court, but this is not a very practical solution when a GP is faced with a conflict between the parents and the medical interests of the child. Discovering the basis for the objection and trying to negotiate an acceptable solution with the parents are important aims. Despite suboptimal health care, the child may be harmed more by removal from the family together with legal proceedings.

The GP and family responsibilities

Some of the most difficult conflicts of interest for GPs arise when the interests of their own families conflict with their professional obligations. Such situations are particularly troublesome because doctors, like any one else in a personal relationship, have primary obligations to seek the best interests of their families.

Case 9.2

Dr Jones has two young children. On Thursdays she works a morning session, leaving at lunchtime to pick her older daughter up from childcare. Today Dr Jones has instructed the practice staff to close off her appointments at 11.15 am so that she can leave early to be present for her daughter's Christmas concert which starts at 12.00.

It is a busy morning in the practice. One of the other doctors on duty has called in sick, and a handful of urgent appointments need to be slotted in. The reception staff want to know if they can add a couple more patients to Dr Jones' list.

There are two primary interests in this case. First, Dr Jones has a primary obligation, as a mother, to care for her children. Whether or not that obligation extends to attending a Christmas concert is arguable, but it is important to acknowledge her legitimate family commitments. Dr Jones has attempted to separate these interests by restricting her surgery times today. Unfortunately, external events have intervened.

Secondly, Dr Jones also has a professional obligation to the patients in her practice. This obligation is strongest for those patients she has already agreed to see, as she has already indicated her willingness to be available for these patients. The extent of Dr Jones' obligations to other patients is a more vexed issue, and will depend on a range of factors, which we will consider below in the section on evaluating conflicts of interest.

Relationships with colleagues

No GP works in isolation from other doctors and health professionals. It is hardly surprising, then, that relationships with colleagues can be problematic at times. Consider the following examples.

Case 9.3

Dr Shah has worked at the Pembroke Crescent Practice in Fetways for several months now.

One evening she was in the local hospital in a nearby town attending a delivery when the senior sister on duty took her aside and mentioned that the doctor on call in casualty that evening had just come in smelling very strongly of alcohol. She was unsure what to do. Dr Shah was not surprised, as it was common knowledge amongst the local medical community that this doctor had a drinking problem.

Dr Shah suggested that they call the medical superintendent in to talk with the doctor and decide whether he was fit to work that evening or not. Unfortunately, when the medical superintendent arrived, he also was drunk and he was unable to make a rational decision about the situation. The medical superintendent then took the sister aside and berated her for her interference. He told he that she should know better than to question the doctor's competence, regardless of whether he'd had any alcohol to drink, and that it was none of her business anyhow.

Dr Shah was appalled by the medical superintendent's actions and decided to take the issue to the next medical staff meeting. At this meeting she was belittled and made to feel that she was young and inexperienced, and that she should not interfere in a situation that required wiser and older heads.

Case 9.4

Dr Schroeder has been working as a locum in a small number of practices for about six months. In one practice, in particular, he has become very uncomfortable with the way that children with chronic asthma are managed. He has strong views that asthma management in children requires a comprehensive approach that includes home monitoring, asthma diaries, and allergy tests. In this practice, doctors do not even take peak flows when the patients come in to see them, relying instead on what appears to Dr Schroeder to be a 'best guess'.

Dr Schroeder only works Saturday mornings in this practice. He acknowledges that his position is short-term and that the patients of the practice are under the long-term care of other GPs. He is reluctant to institute asthma management programmes with the children he sees, because their regular doctors will not follow up the programmes. His solution is to make no changes to the patients' management, and just to make some suggestions in the case notes about future management options for them. He couches these suggestions as ideas from another doctor who has just cast their eyes over this particular patient, without necessarily doing much. He does not mention the possibility of different management to the patients at all.

Medical misconduct of the type described in these cases seems to be a particularly difficult issue for doctors to deal with. Some writers suggest that most cases of medical misconduct are ignored by the profession (Rhodes and Cohen 2001). Colleagues are often slow to act because they fear the consequences both for themselves and for the doctor whose conduct is in question. Doctors may fear being ostracized, threatened, or losing their job if they question a colleague's competence. And, they may not be confident that the doctor will actually be helped if his misconduct is reported (Rhodes and Cohen 2001, p. 217).

GPs must remember that their primary concern in these situations is the best interests of patients, rather than a secondary interest in the good name of the profession or in their own welfare. The General Medical Council is clear on this:

> You must protect patients from risk of harm posed by another doctor's, or other health care professional's, conduct, performance or health, including problems arising from alcohol or other substance abuse. The safety of patients must come first at all times. Where there are serious concerns about a colleague's performance, health or conduct, it is essential that steps are taken without delay to investigate the concerns to establish whether they are well-founded, and to protect patients.

GMC 2001, para 26

Even with such clear advice, deciding exactly how to intervene in such situations can be very difficult, and a careful evaluation, perhaps with the aid of an experienced colleague, is required. If a GP is concerned about the competence of a colleague, the first step is always to be as sure of the facts as possible. Having collected as much information as possible, the GP should bring their concerns to an appropriate person in a position of authority, such as the medical director, nursing director or chief executive, or the director of public health, or an officer of the medical committee (GMC 2001).

For more minor situations of conflict, such as that experienced by Dr Schroeder, it may be possible to address concerns with the doctor personally, or within the practice. Despite his temporary status in the practice, Dr Schroeder's primary obligation is to the patients he sees. There is also nothing wrong with telling patients that there is a difference of opinion about how certain conditions should be managed, and allowing them to raise these issues with their regular GP (Osgood *et al.* 2000). This can usually be achieved without making negative comments to patients about other GPs' abilities or decisions.

Relationships with pharmaceutical companies

The relationship between the pharmaceutical industry and doctors has become a source of considerable tension and controversy. Concerns about the impact of the relationship between drug companies and GPs on patient care arise for a number of reasons (Komesaroff and Kerridge 2002). First, there is concern that relations between drug companies and doctors may function to advance commercial interests and doctors' self-interest, rather than patient care or research. Secondly, there is the possibility that involvement of the pharmaceutical industry in research can lead to biased reporting of research results. Finally, there is concern that drug advertising and promotion may influence doctors' prescribing decisions inappropriately.

For GPs the most immediate of these three issues is the last one. Many (if not most) doctors believe that they make prescribing decisions based on their clinical experience and the scientific evidence. They ignore, however, the subtle effects of advertising on their prescribing behaviour. In fact, as Komesaroff and Kerridge note, there is considerable evidence that advertising by drug companies does affect doctors' decision-making:

> Contact with drug company representatives leads to prescribing more of their drugs; physicians exposed to advertising are more likely to accept commercial rather than well-established scientific views; and drug company advertising is associated with an inability of some physicians to identify wrong claims and propensity to engage in non-rational prescribing behaviour.
>
> (Komesaroff and Kerridge 2002, p. 119)

Gift giving and support for travel and conference attendance have similarly been shown to influence doctors' prescribing behaviour. For example, Chren and Landefeld (1994) found that doctors who received honoraria from drug companies to speak at meetings were 21 times more likely to ask that the companies' products be included in their hospital's formulary.

Pharmaceutical company sponsorship of scientific meetings and continuing medical education activities poses particular difficulties for GPs. Doctors and drug companies both stand to gain from such activities; educational events, particularly, may be expensive to mount and sponsorship can provide a welcome injection of funds. However, there is clear evidence here, as elsewhere, that drug company sponsorship of educational events increases prescriptions of drugs marketed by that company (Komesaroff and Kerridge 2002).

Those who are against drug advertising, in all its forms, argue that the evidence above leads to the conclusion that drug promotion can result in individual patients receiving treatment that is not warranted. In addition, they point to the high cost of pharmaceuticals and the impact that unnecessary prescribing has on the overall cost of health care (Katz *et al.* 2003).

Against such evidence of the negative impact of pharmaceutical advertising, many GPs argue that the information provided by drug companies is helpful and that they rely on it to make their own independent assessments (Weber 2001). Even if they accept that support from pharmaceutical companies does have an impact on their prescribing habits, they may argue that the outcome is rarely detrimental to patients. Many patients will actually benefit from having a particular drug prescribed. There is also the argument that some activities sponsored by pharmaceutical companies are worthwhile in their own right as they provide opportunities for education and exchange of ideas that would otherwise not be available.

Consider, for example, the situation of Dr Chu below.

Case 9.5

With 25% of his patients HIV positive, Dr Chu has developed an interest in HIV medicine, particularly in the management of AIDS in primary care settings. He works with a team of nurses, health visitors, psychologists, and social workers with expertise in this area.

Once a month, Dr Chu hosts an HIV case conference in his practice. It is a breakfast meeting attended by staff in the practice and surrounding practices who have an interest in the care of patients with HIV/AIDS. The breakfast is provided by Links–Howard, a pharmaceutical company which produces a range of drugs used in the treatment of HIV/AIDS. One of the Links–Howard pharmaceutical representatives also attends these meetings.

The meetings usually begin informally as the participants eat breakfast together. They then spend about half an hour either discussing general treatment and management issues or one participant will bring a difficult case to the meeting. Dr Chu allows the Links–Howard representative to speak for up to 10 minutes at the end of each meeting.

Links–Howard also regularly offers to pay for Dr Chu's attendance at conferences related to HIV/AIDS. About once per year, Dr Chu accepts Links–Howard's invitation, usually to attend a conference in the United States.

Dr Chu probably believes that his contact with Links–Howard in its various forms has little or no impact on his practice. In particular, he may feel that his expertise in HIV medicine allows him to judge impartially the information that the Links–Howard representatives offer him and his colleagues. The empirical evidence set out above can make uncomfortable reading for GPs like Dr Chu who believe that their own clinical judgement is not influenced by their contact with the pharmaceutical industry.

Dr Chu's most powerful reason for maintaining his contact with Links–Howard is likely to be that he feels the breakfast meetings achieve a great deal of good, with relatively little likelihood of harm. The scientific updates provide an easy way for staff to increase their knowledge and skills and the monthly case conferences allow the practice to review and enhance its quality of care. Dr Chu may also believe that providing breakfast is a simple courtesy to people who are adding an extra activity on to already busy lives.

These arguments for and against accepting gifts, money, and sponsorship from drug companies make evaluation of conflicts of interest in this arena particularly difficult. A similar set of issues arises for GPs who accept payments for enrolling patients into clinical trials.

Inducements to participate in research

Case 9.6

Mr Shawlands is approached by his GP, Dr Grainger, to take part in a clinical trial. Dr Grainger tells Mr Shawlands that involvement in the trial will mean that his hypertension is monitored carefully for the duration of the trial, and he implies that this might not happen otherwise. He also suggests that Mr Shawlands is doing something worthwhile for society if he agrees to take part, just as Dr Grainger's participation is also helping the advancement of science. Mr Shawlands agrees to participate, mainly because he admires Dr Grainger, and likes to think they are both helping a good cause.

Mr Shawlands finds his involvement in the trial rather inconvenient, as it involves a number of extra trips to the surgery. Sometimes he needs to take time off work to attend.

About halfway through the trial Mr Shawlands learns from a friend that Dr Grainger is receiving £50 for every patient he enrols in the trial.

There are a number of ethical issues in this case. As with the previous examples, Dr Grainger's primary obligation is to further the best interests of his patients, with or without their participation in any research. The suggestion that participation in the trial will secure regular monitoring of Mr Shaw's blood pressure that would not otherwise be available is of concern, suggesting that routine care is not of a high standard. We might also be concerned about the extent to which Mr Shawlands has given his informed consent to participate in this trial, on the basis of the way Dr Grainger appears to have described the trial to him. Finally, the inconvenience Mr Shawlands is experiencing does not seem trivial and it is important to explore the possibility that Mr Shawlands is actually being harmed by his involvement in the trial.

The ethical concerns expressed above do not address at all the conflict of interests that Dr Grainger has in taking part in this research. In the next section we set out a number of strategies for evaluating such conflicts.

Evaluating conflicts of interest

The problem with conflicts of interest is not that they exist, but the extent to which they engender morally unacceptable conduct. We can evaluate the moral acceptability of a conflict of interests by considering four components of the conflict:

(a) How avoidable the conflict is.

(b) The legitimacy of the interests in the conflict.

(c) The likelihood that professional judgement will be influenced, or appear to be influenced by secondary interests.

(d) The seriousness of the impact on the primary interest (Thompson 1993; Goold 2000).

How avoidable is this conflict of interests?

Some conflicts of interest are inevitable. For example, the means through which GPs are paid inevitably generates some conflict of interests, whether the system used is a capitation scheme (which may encourage under-servicing) or fee-for-service payments (which may encourage over-servicing). Dr Shah and Dr Schroeder also can not avoid their conflicts: they are bound by the obligations to patients to address the medical misconduct they observe.

On the other hand, some conflicts can be avoided. Consider, for example, the following scenario.

Case 9.7

Every year Dr Carter takes his family on an overseas holiday, often to Australia, where his wife has relatives. He believes that this break is essential to his health and well-being. To maximize the time abroad, Dr Carter generally arrives back in the UK on the morning he is due to start work again. He showers at the airport and drives directly to his inner London practice to start work at 9.00 am.

Dr Carter's colleagues and staff are beginning to express their annoyance with his behaviour. For the last couple of years, there have been complaints from patients that Dr Carter seems unable to concentrate on their problems during his first days back. Dr Carter, however, insists that he is fine and that he needs every minute of his time away.

In this situation, Dr Carter has a conflict of interests between his primary obligations to his patients and his colleagues and his secondary interest in a relaxing and satisfying holiday. However, this conflict is not inevitable: Dr Carter could arrange his time such that he returned to the UK one or two days earlier, thus mitigating the worst effects of the long-haul flight from Australia. Generally speaking, conflicts of interest that are avoidable require a higher level of justification than those that are unavoidable.

How legitimate are the interests?

Some interests are more legitimate or justifiable than others. There is never any doubt that primary interests such as patient welfare, the integrity of research, education, and high standards for the profession are legitimate interests for doctors to have. In a similar way, certain interests such as a desire to harm patients, or to undermine credible research, are always illegitimate. However, many secondary interests, while not in and of themselves illegitimate, can become unjustifiable under certain circumstances. In our example above, no one would question that Dr Carter has a legitimate interest in his own welfare, which he expresses by regular holidays in a location that he finds relaxing and satisfying. Nonetheless, the extent to which he pursues this interest arguably makes it unjustifiable.

The RCGP/GPC (BMA) guidelines on financial and commercial dealings in general practice include a number of examples of circumstances in which a GP's secondary interest in financial gain is unjustifiable:

(a) Accepting a fee from a specialist or clinic for a referral without informing the patient.

(b) Abuse of funds provided for practice expenses or patient treatment.

(c) Defrauding the NHS or any organization you work for.

(d) Exerting pressure on patients to enter a nursing home which you own (RCGP/GPC (BMA) 2002, p. 45).

In addition, the guidelines also note that accepting gifts and hospitality is an area of particular concern and suggest that GPs limit the gifts they accept to trivial ones.

How likely is it that professional judgement will be influenced, or appear to be influenced, by secondary interests?

The likelihood that a GP's professional judgement will be influenced in a conflict of interests is related to a number of factors (Thompson 1993). First, there is the size of the inducement being offered. The greater the personal benefit to the GP, for example, the more likely it is that it will influence his primary interest in his patients' well-being. All other things being equal, the conflict of interests that Dr Chu faces by regularly accepting sponsorship to attend overseas conferences is more serious than that faced by his colleagues who merely eat breakfasts supplied by the pharmaceutical company.

Secondly, the scope of the conflict is also relevant to the likelihood of influence, in particular as it relates to the nature of the relationship that has created the conflict. For example, a long-standing and close relationship in which a GP benefits many times from, say, continued support by a pharmaceutical company is more troubling that once-off gifts. The reasons for this are obvious. Over time, continuing relationships come to generate their own momentum; the GP may enjoy his contact with particular pharmaceutical company representatives and value the relationships he forms for themselves. In addition, he may come to depend on the regular gifts, money, or support offered by the company. Dr Chu is at risk of being in this situation. Links–Howard regularly sponsors his breakfast meetings, and Dr Chu may doubt that he would be able to sustain this activity without the support of the company.

The amount of independence the GP is able to exercise with respect to the judgements he makes is also relevant in a conflict of interests. For example, if there are practice standards that restrict the drugs a GP can prescribe, then that GP is less open to influence by contact with pharmaceutical representatives than one who has total discretion about prescribing practices.

How serious is the impact of the conflict on the primary interest?

In evaluating a conflict of interests, it is important to review how seriously any primary interest will be affected. There is often a spectrum of seriousness, ranging from no likelihood of influence (or even a benefit) through to quite serious consequences. For example, consider the possibility that Dr Chu changes his medication regime for specific patients based on his most recent attendance at a conference sponsored by Links–Howard. The change may improve the quality of life of his patients at no greater cost. Alternatively, there may be no improvement, or perhaps an increase in annoying side-effects. The new drug may also be more expensive, resulting in increased out-ofpocket expenses for his patients.

Beyond direct impacts on the care of individual patients, Dr Chu needs to think about the more generalized effects of secondary interests. There may be increased costs for the health system overall if he prescribes more costly drugs. Dr Chu may also want to consider the impact that it might have on his patients more generally, should it become known that he is supported by Links–Howard.

Dealing with conflicts of interest

This last point leads naturally to a consideration of remedies for conflict of interest. The remedy most often proposed for conflicts of interest is disclosure to all people who might be affected by the conflict. This gives people who are likely to be affected by the GP's conflict of interests opportunity to draw their own conclusions about the likely impact on their well-being. Dr Chu could begin to deal with his conflict of interest by including in his practice information leaflet a note stating that the practice receives support from the pharmaceutical company, Howard–Links. He could briefly describe the forms that this sponsorship takes and indicate that he is prepared to answer questions about the sponsorship.

Merely disclosing a conflict of interests is rarely a remedy in its own right. 'Disclosing a conflict only reveals a problem, without providing any guidance for resolving it' (Thompson 1993). In fact, all disclosure may do, in the short-term, is to increase anxiety, which can undermine trust in the medical profession. Patients who are informed that drug company promotions take place in their practice may question whether other factors also shape the decisions and advice they receive. Similarly, Dr Jones may decide to see an extra patient before she leaves, and to inform the patient as she enters the consulting room that she is in a hurry to get to her daughter's concert. Disclosing information to patients in this situation can do a great deal of harm to the doctor–patient relationship.

The dangers inherent in merely disclosing a conflict of interests do not imply that doctors should keep such conflicts secret. Rather, making others aware of the conflict is really just the first step in addressing the conflict appropriately. The next step is to carefully evaluate the conflict, and identify its various components. Thoughtful analysis of the avoidability and legitimacy of the conflict, as well as the likelihood of undue influence and the seriousness of the impact, may lead to a number of outcomes. The conflict may be deemed to be avoidable. Dr Carter's conflict of interest, for example, can be resolved if he returns to the UK from his holiday 24 hours earlier. Dr Chu can refuse to accept sponsorship to travel to conferences at Links–Howard's expense. And, Dr Grainger can request that the payment for his participation in the clinical trial reflect more accurately the time and resources he puts into the trial. Alternatively, analysis of the conflict may suggest that the secondary interest is illegitimate. Some secondary interests can be dismissed as unethical immediately. Interests which may lead to harm and lack of respect for patients, or which may undermine the integrity of research, fall into this category.

Some conflicts of interest are neither avoidable, nor totally unjustifiable. We then need to think about the likelihood of undue influence and the seriousness of the impact. The onus here is on showing that secondary interests—for example, financial gain, prestige, or public recognition—will *not* exert an undue influence on primary interests such as patient care or research integrity, and that the impact such secondary interests have will be minor.

Occasionally, GPs will encounter situations either of conflict between primary interests or where secondary interests are justifiably powerful. Dr Jones' dilemma concerning attending her daughter's Christmas concert is such a situation. In these situations, the GP may need to recognize that her loyalties are unavoidably divided and that she can not get it completely right. O'Neill, writing in a slightly different context, suggests that:

> Where existing realities may force hard choices, it may be impossible to
> meet all of the various requirements . . . The unmeetable requirement may
> have 'remainders' and remainders are often viewed as calling for expressions
> of attitudes such as regret or remorse . . . More active responses might
> include expressions of apology, commitment to reform, the provision of
> compensation, forms of restitution, making good, and the like.

(O'Neill 2001, p. 22)

Just because we cannot reconcile conflicts of interest on all occasions does not mean that we should avoid choosing one over the other in individual instances. GPs may need to make a choice, and note that the choice is imperfect.

One solution that is not likely to work in a conflict of interests is keeping the conflict secret. GPs who are tempted to keep conflicts of interest hidden should bear in mind what is likely to happen should patients and other interested parties learn that the conflict has been concealed. If patients learn that their doctor's secondary interests, such as financial gain, have influenced decisions regarding their treatment, and that the doctor has taken steps to keep this information secret, this is far more likely to harm the doctor–patient relationship. Consider, for example, the situation of Mr Shawlands and his participation in Dr Grainger's clinical trial. Mr Shawlands is likely to feel annoyed when he learns that Dr Grainger has a financial interest in the trial. It makes little difference if Dr Grainger's principal motive for enrolling patients in the trial is to advance the state of scientific knowledge. The appearance of a conflict of interests is enough to generate concern, and the fact that Dr Grainger's financial gain has been kept secret from his patients can only exacerbate Mr Shawlands' loss of faith in Dr Grainger.

It can be difficult for GPs caught up in conflicts of interest to stand back and evaluate their involvement impartially. For this reason, at the very least, any GP involved in a conflict of interests should seek advice from an experienced and independent colleague. In some cases, contact with the GP's medical defence organization or the General Medical Council may be prudent. In addition, there are certain situations in which review and authorization by independent organizations is required. For example, GPs who take part in research may only accept payments that have been approved by a Research Ethics Committee (Royal College of General Practitioners/General Practitioners Committee (British Medical Association) 2002).

Conclusion

In this chapter we have explored a wide range of ethical problems that can grouped together as examples of conflicts of interest. We have suggested that thinking about these conflicts as clashes between primary and secondary interests is helpful. We have also indicated that such conflicts can be evaluated by considering the avoidability and legitimacy of the conflict, as well as the likelihood of undue influence and the seriousness of the impact. Disclosure is generally an important first step in beginning to address a conflict of interests, but often it will not be the sole action a GP needs to take.

References

Chren, M.M. and Landefeld, S. (1994). Physicians' behaviour and their interactions with drug companies. *Journal of the American Medical Association* **271**, 684–9.

General Medical Council. (2001). *Good medical practice.* General Medical Council, London.

Goold, S.D. (2000). Conflicts of interest and obligation. In Sugarman, J. (ed.) *20 common problems—ethics in primary care*, pp. 93–101. McGraw-Hill, New York, NY.

Kassirer, J.P. and Angell, M. (1993). Financial conflicts of interest in biomedical research. *New England Journal of Medicine* **329**, 570–1.

Katz, D., Caplan, A.L., and Merz, J.F. (2003). All gifts large and small: toward an understanding of the ethics of pharmaceutical industry giving. *American Journal of Bioethics* **3**(3), 39–46.

Komesaroff, P.A. and Kerridge, I.H. (2002). Ethical issues concerning the relationship between medical practitioners and the pharmaceutical industry. *Medical Journal of Australia* **176**, 118–21.

Lemmens, T. and Singer, P.A. (1998). Bioethics for clinicians: conflicts of interest in research, education and patient care. *Canadian Medical Association Journal* **159**, 960–5.

O'Neill, O. (2001). Practical principles and practical judgement. *Hasting Center Report* **31**(4), 15–23.

Osgood, B.S. Krasny, A.J., and Emanuel, L.L. (2000). Consultation and referral. In Sugarman, J. (ed.) *20 common problems—ethics in primary care*, pp. 103–15. McGraw-Hill, New York, NY.

Pellegrino, E.D. (1987). Altruism, self-interest, and medical ethics. *Journal of the American Medical Association* **258**, 1939–40.

Pellegrino, E.D. (1994). Self-interest, the physician's duties and medical ethics: a philosophical and theological challenge. In Campbell, C.S. and Lustig, B.A. (ed.) *Duties to others*, pp. 125–41. Kluwer Academic Publishers, Netherlands.

Rhodes, R. and Cohen, N. (2001). Abusing alcohol or drugs—Commentaries. In Kushner, T.K. and Thomasma, D.C. (ed.) *Ward ethics. Dilemmas for medical students and doctors in training*, pp. 216–22. Cambridge University Press, Cambridge.

Royal College of General Practitioners/General Practitioners Committee (British Medical Association). (2002). *Good medical practice for general practitioners*. Royal College of General Practitioners, London.

Thompson, D.F. (1993). Understanding financial conflicts of interest. *New England Journal of Medicine* **329**, 573–6.

Weber, J. (2001). Commentary—Conflicts of interest. In Kushner, T.K. and Thomasma, D.C. (ed.) *Ward ethics. Dilemmas for medical students and doctors in training*, pp. 208–10. Cambridge University Press, Cambridge.

Further reading

Erde, E.L. (1996). Conflicts of interest in medicine: A philosophical and ethical morphology. In Spece, R.G., Shimm, D.S., and Buchanan, A.E. (ed.) *Conflicts of interest in clinical practice and research* pp. 12–41. Oxford University Press, New York, NY.

Hazard, G.C. (1996). Conflicts of interest in the classic professions. In Spece, R.G., Shimm, D.S., and Buchanan, A.E. (ed.) *Conflicts of interest in clinical practice and research* pp. 85–104. Oxford University Press, New York, NY.

Lemmens, T. and Singer, P.A. (1998). Bioethics for clinicians: Conflicts of interest in research, education and patient care. *Canadian Medical Association Journal* **159**, 960–5.

Rodwin, M.A. (1993). *Medicine, money, and morals: physicians' conflicts of interest*. Oxford University Press, New York, NY.

Chapter 10

On being a good doctor: virtues in general practice

Introduction

In 2002, the *British Medical Journal* ran a series of articles on the question: 'What is a good doctor?' The issue clearly struck a chord in the journal's readership, as evidenced by the flurry of letters in response. The journal and its readers also recognized that they were not the only ones interested in the question of what makes a good doctor. Patients are just as interested in the answer to this question, not least because a number of recent cases in Britain have eroded public confidence in medicine.

Just what is a good doctor? And, more specifically, what is a good general practitioner? This chapter explores this question, drawing on virtue theory, a branch of ethics that is explicitly concerned with human character and ideas about goodness (and badness) in human beings.

What is different about a virtues approach to ethics in general practice?

So far in this book we have given an account of ethics in general practice that has emphasized 'doing the right thing', for example in the realm of doing what's best for the patient, or respecting patient autonomy. But, some philosophers do not think that all of ethical practice can be explained by focusing just on what we do. The kinds of people we are, the character traits we have, our intentions and motives, are all important for a complete account of what living an ethically good life involves. And some of these concepts are hard to capture within a definition of ethics that concentrates exclusively on what we do.

Here are two simple examples by way of illustration.

Case 10.1

Dr Bowler is leaving his surgery late Friday evening. It's been a long day and he's tired, grumpy, and he has a headache. If he could wave a magic wand he would walk out the door of his practice and never comes back. As he's leaving, the phone rings. He hesitates and then picks it up. Mrs Lonsdale is at the other end, worried about her son James. Dr Bowler's demeanour is polite, calm, and focused. He asks a few questions and decides that he really ought to see James.

Dr Bowler's behaviour is exactly what we would expect of a morally excellent doctor, yet his actions here are not taken after a lengthy period of self-reflection during which he is able to weigh up what the best thing to do in this situation might be. Dr Bowler responds *intuitively* with patience and fortitude. He does not let his tiredness or frustration show and he treats Mrs Lonsdale exactly as he would have done had she been the first patient he saw after his annual holiday. We probably think that this is how Dr Bowler usually behaves (even though we may be at a loss to understand how he achieves this). Somehow or other, he has learnt to respond to situations like this in a morally exemplary manner.

Now, consider a rather different situation. The example is adapted from Veatch (1985).

Case 10.2

Dr Imogen Jones joined the Westminster Surgery in Bath five years after graduating with honours from medical school. She appears to be an exemplary doctor. Her technical knowledge and skills are superb and she knows how to use them appropriately in a general practice setting. The patients value her greatly: she listens carefully, is respectful, and offers advice judiciously. What's more, she is considerate and thoughtful in her dealings with the staff of the practice, while being appropriately assertive. One evening Dr Bowler invites Imogen and her husband, Hugh, over for a meal. After dinner, talk turns to why people become doctors and how they get to be the sort of doctors they are. Dr Bowler rehearses his own reasons for studying medicine, mumbling something about wanting to help people, while doing something scientific. He mentions his belief that people are 'all the same, underneath' and says that he tries to treat patients as equals. "Although I've got a lot more skills in some areas than a lot of the patients, they've got a lot of skills that I haven't got. I mean, if a man is a plumber I wouldn't know how to begin to do a drain out, would I?"

When Dr Bowler asks Imogen about her reasons for becoming a doctor, he is stunned by the reply: "I only became a doctor to make money, and that still really determines how I do things. I realized early on that doctors who appear kind, thoughtful, and considerate, who try to fit in with their colleagues, who communicate well, do better. If I didn't think it was in my interests, I would give up being nice to patients tomorrow."

There is something deeply disturbing about Imogen, about a doctor who does all the right things, but for reasons that appear, intuitively, to be wrong.

Both examples illustrate that our attitudes, motives, characters, and fundamental dispositions to behave in certain ways are all morally relevant. Virtue theory is concerned with just these issues. It offers a vehicle to incorporate ideas about character and motives into an account of ethics in general practice.

What is virtue ethics?

Virtue ethics is concerned with the kinds of abilities and attitudes we need to have to be able to act morally. The focus, as we noted above, is on character and therefore on the way in which morally good people respond to situations. Virtue theorists hold the view that what makes an action right is that it is done by someone of virtuous character. In one fell swoop this simple observation shifts our attention quite dramatically from the things that a person does to what that person is like—their character, their settled ways of doing things, their personality traits.

In a general practice context, a virtue ethics approach asks: 'What kind of person is a morally good GP?' At an intuitive level, we all can answer this question by listing off character traits that we think are worthwhile or virtuous. We may think of things such as honesty, trustworthiness, benevolence, respectfulness, courage, and integrity. What makes these characteristics virtues is that they share a focus on human flourishing; they contribute to the capacity for humans to live well together. The good GP contributes to human flourishing in a range of ways but, most particularly, through serving her patients' medical interests. Trustworthiness, benevolence, respectfulness, and fairness in dealing with others all contribute to this end. In the following section of this chapter we want to consider one more virtue which we think is especially important in a general practice context: the virtue of compassion.

Compassion

GPs frequently encounter suffering in their work and they have many ways to deal with it. Some GPs practise a form of 'detached concern', building a barrier between themselves and their patients that recognizes the pain but refuses to let it touch them (Brody 1998). Less commonly, there are GPs whose experience of their patients' misfortunes almost seems to mimic the patients' suffering. Then there are a small group of doctors whose defence mechanisms are so well developed that they no longer see suffering at all.

Such responses are not part of the practice of the virtuous doctor. Rather, the virtuous doctor responds to suffering with compassion. We think that compassion is a particularly important virtue for general practice, because it offers GPs a way to manage their ongoing contact with apparently inexplicable instances of illness, suffering, death and misfortune, *and* the pull of those instances on their emotions.

Just what is involved in being a compassionate GP? We suggest that compassion has four characteristics (Nussbaum 1996; Blum 1997).

The compassionate GP focuses on people who are suffering

Compassion is a response to pain or suffering in others. The person for whom compassion is felt must be suffering a harm, be in some difficulty, or be in danger. The suffering also needs to be reasonably serious or, at least, not trivial. Compassion is typically evoked when we see death, pain, or serious illness, all things that are part and parcel of the GP's daily work.

It is important to note here that the GP who feels compassion does not simply accept other people's judgements about the seriousness of their suffering. The compassionate GP has her own point of view on the suffering she sees. She doesn't necessarily agree to see things as her patient sees them; in fact, she may ascribe a rather different value to what she sees happening to a patient. This independence of judgement can cut two ways. First, the GP may not necessarily think her patient's misfortune is as significant as he thinks it is. For example, when otherwise fit and healthy John comes to see his GP complaining loudly of a sore throat of 24 hours duration, we hardly expect the GP's response to be compassion. On the other hand, a compassionate GP can also 'feel for' the patient who seems unaware that his situation warrants compassion. Imagine an elderly man caring, with little support, for his dying wife. The GP can see that the husband's physical and psychological health is suffering; yet, the man refuses to accept help and will not even acknowledge that what he is doing is out of the ordinary. Rather, he sees this as 'just doing what has to be done'. He may not thinks his situation makes him worthy of compassion; we would probably agree with the GP that it does.

Compassion involves imagining what the suffering must be like

Compassion is obviously much more than just an attitude directed toward a person who is suffering, because indifference or curiosity are also attitudes that can be directed at people who suffer. We do occasionally meet health professionals who seem to adopt this disengaged, but interested, attitude towards patients who are clearly in psychological or physical pain. We may wonder whether there is something 'missing' in their attitude or approach to patients; that something is compassion.

Being compassionate means that we actively try to imagine what it must be like to be suffering as this patient is suffering. This is not the same as 'identifying' with the patient, where the emphasis is rather more on what I would feel if I were in that situation. Identifying involves blurring the boundaries between the GP and the patient such that the GP can no longer really tell where the patient's experience ends and the GP's begins. Nor does the capacity to imagine the other's condition require that a GP have experienced in the past what his patient is experiencing now, although prior experience may certainly help us to imagine what it is like for other people.

Martha Nussbaum frames this imaginative reconstruction in a rather different way and calls it 'a judgement of *similar possibilities*' (Nussbaum 1996, p. 34). She emphasizes that this does not mean that a compassionate GP should suffer *with* patients. Rather, the GP always sees herself as separate from the patient, while recognizing that the pain, illness, misfortune that the patient is experiencing could, under different conditions, happen to her.

The fact that compassion judges another's suffering to be possible for oneself is what sets it apart from the response of intellectual curiosity or indifference. The compassionate onlooker knows that goods such as food, health, freedom, etc., *do* matter, and that none of us are immune from having these goods taken away from us. Compassion is one of those virtues that help us to cross class, nationality, race, and gender boundaries; the compassionate person 'assumes these different positions in imagination, and comes to see the obstacles to flourishing faced by human beings in these many concrete situations' (Nussbaum 1996, p. 51).

Being able to accept other people's suffering as possibilities for ourselves is what allows compassion to be a 'bridge between the individual and the community' (Nussbaum 1996, p. 28). That bridge involves regarding the other people as human beings, like us, and it means acknowledging that there is some sense in which we are equal. It is exemplified in the way Dr Bowler, at the beginning of this chapter, attempted to define his relationship with his patients: 'we're all the

same, underneath'. It may help to see why this sense of shared human-
ity is important to compassion if we think about situations in which
it is absent. It is hard to imagine feeling compassion for someone
whom we regard as superior to or above ourselves in some way, and it
is pity, rather than compassion, that we feel for someone whom we
think is inferior to or below us in some way. In both cases, we deem
the other person 'fundamentally different' from ourselves.

Because compassion has this quality of imaginative reconstruction
of others' experiences, people who find it hard to imagine other ways
of seeing, doing, and being things tend to be less compassionate. It is
also why some doctors will say that, as they become older, they feel the
pull of compassion more deeply. This may be, at least in part, because
their broader life experiences can not but create a greater awareness of
what life is like for other people.

Compassion involves active concern for the well-being of others

Compassion makes no sense unless it is tied to caring about and, usually,
trying to alleviate the suffering that we observe. The compassionate
doctor does much more than acknowledge and interpret her patients'
suffering. She also cares that they are suffering and she wants to do something about that suffering. Often, there will be much that she can do.
She can attempt to find the cause of the pain, discomfort, and suffering;
she can offer treatment and advice for self-management. Here, the
motive or her actions will not be primarily that it makes her feel better
(although that may well be the case), but that it will improve things for her
patients.

Compassion is a driver for beneficent actions towards patients. We
can see very clearly here the difference between the action of doing
good and the intentions and motives that drive those actions. Imogen
Jones behaves beneficently—she acts for the good of her patients—but
she lacks compassion, for her motives ultimately concern only herself.

Ironically, compassion has a particularly important role to play
when we can not manage to alleviate suffering. The compassionate
person is optimistic: she continues to hope that something will work
to lessen the suffering, or to allay the fears. Merely being with people

in their suffering can make a difference, and many patients will testify to how much it did help to have their GP just 'being with them'. Moreover, because a compassionate doctor continues to care in the face of apparent defeat, she is more open to unexpected or unlikely sources of relief for patients. Compassion carries with it a sense of never giving up. This does not mean refusing to recognize terminal illness or endlessly striving for a cure, but rather never giving up on the patient.

Compassion is an enduring emotion

Compassion is not a transient attitude which is here today, gone tomorrow. Like other virtues, it is characterized by its enduring quality; it is a trait that we develop and exhibit over a long period of time. Again, it is easy to see why this is the case if one considers expressions of concern that are more fleeting. The momentary twinges of conscience some of us feel when we contemplate the victims of an earthquake or a famine on the other side of the world may indicate our concern for the plight of others. However, unless those twinges develop into something more lasting, we would hardly describe our response as compassion.

Limits to compassion

Compassion, when understood wrongly or practised inappropriately, can actually cause harm. Patients may be harmed by a GP who is over-compassionate, as this may encourage the patient to focus too much on his illness. GPs may be harmed, if compassion leads to an exclusive focus on one patient's suffering to the detriment of other patients, or if it blinds the GP to a more balanced way of seeing things. Like all of the virtues, compassion is not a virtue to be practised in isolation. In particular, compassion must be tempered with the following:

(a) Respectfulness—to maintain a sense of patients as independent and able to chart their own course.

(b) Justice—to ensure that all patients are treated fairly, with due consideration given to each person who needs it.

(c) Beneficence—to keep what is in the patient's best interests in the forefront at all times and, in particular, to ensure that knowledge and reason prevail.

Medical vices

If there can be virtues in and for general practice, there can also be vices. A number of writers also refer to vices in medicine, generally by way of contrast with the virtues (Drane 1994). One way to frame a discussion of the vices is in terms of commitments. Medical vices are character traits that accompany the wrong kinds of ultimate commitments: to money, to power, to science, or to self. We will look at each of these briefly.

There is a long, and sometimes unpleasant, history behind descriptions of doctors as 'only in it for the money', but the topic is canvassed only rarely in medical ethics textbooks. Imogen Jones, at the beginning of this chapter, is unusual in her forthright commitment to money. To understand what disturbs us about Imogen's position, we need to go back to our definition of a virtue. The problem with being ultimately committed to acquiring money for oneself is that this is unlikely to be compatible with the ends of medicine, in terms of healing or care for patients. The doctor committed ultimately to money ceases to care for patients when there is no economic benefit for herself. In a similar way, an ultimate commitment to power runs counter to empowering patients or even to working productively in a team with other health professionals.

An ultimate commitment to science might seem a somewhat strange inclusion in a list of vices. What could be wrong with being committed to a medicine that is practised scientifically? The problem is, again, the notion of an ultimate commitment. The GP who is ultimately committed to science risks losing interest in patients when science alone can provide no biological remedies. This is a perilous route for general practice, for, as we have discussed previously, there is much of general practice care that does not turn on scientific evidence and proven treatments. Nor can GPs expect even to be able to offer an effective remedy for all the problems they meet.

Finally, there is the question of having an ultimate commitment to self. We have explored the role of self-interest in our chapter on conflicts of interest. There we suggested that GPs who pursue secondary interests such as personal gain, power, or prestige risk damaging the relationship of trust that ought to exist between them and their patients. At the end of the moral day, it is Imogen Jones' selfishness, her ultimate commitment to self, which most disturbs us. Someone who is turned in on herself can not really be trusted to pursue the best interests of patients in her care.

Why do we need a focus on the virtues in medicine?

We have suggested that compassion is an important virtue for general practice. Along with other virtues, it implies a different way to think about moral goods in general practice. Before we conclude our discussion of the virtues, we want to make a few points about the special value of a virtue ethics approach (Pellegrino 1995).

Some writers, such as Edmund Pellegrino, think that we need an emphasis on virtue as a corrective to some current morally questionable practices in medicine—refusing to treat patients with AIDS, turning away the poor, complying with early discharge rules when it is medically inappropriate, medical entrepreneurialism. Perhaps if we concentrated more on selecting, training, and encouraging doctors to be virtuous, we would have less of these practices.

Others argue that we need to emphasize the virtues because of the specialization and bureaucratization of medicine (May 1994). These factors have meant that we now see very little of what an individual practitioner does, where once the doctor's work was more open to scrutiny. The argument here is clearest if we contrast, say, the practice of a specialist vascular surgeon working in a large city today with that of a general practitioner based in a small rural village fifty years ago. Fifty years ago, an efficient grapevine would have ensured that the country doctor's successes and failures were more widely known than the vascular surgeon's could ever be today. In addition, the country doctor would be the sole recipient of any blame or praise, that is now dispersed widely in institutions rather than attributed to individuals. A focus on virtue can help protect us against the self-interested physician, who, in a smaller world, would have been scrutinized carefully by a watchful community.

Thirdly, focusing on virtues such as compassion reminds us that good general practice involves far more than technical skill. A virtuous doctor is certainly technically competent: she displays the skills of an applied scientist in combining her clinical expertise with familiarity and appropriate application of the best available evidence. But a virtuous doctor is also more than a sophisticated diagnostic therapeutic machine. A virtuous doctor is humane: he displays the personal qualities that human beings need to assist people in their suffering.

Finally, a virtue ethics approach also encourages us to think about how we become the sort of people we are. Although virtues are, in some ways, intuitive, they are not things 'we find ourselves with, but something we construct over a lifetime' (Drane 1994, pp. 294–5). The virtues are acquired human qualities, learnt and practised in what we do and how we think about our actions. This component to our description of a virtue suggests that we can learn to be certain kinds of people; we can try to develop certain ways of responding to things and to limit other ways. When an experienced GP says: "One of the things I've had to learn over the years is to control my impatience when people don't catch on as quickly as I do", we see virtue as a practised skill in action.

This notion of the virtues as acquired human qualities also opens up a discussion about the close two-way relationship between character development and the social and cultural environment. The way in which character is formed is obviously influenced by the social settings in which people live. So, how we educate doctors is important, not only for the technical knowledge and skills that are learnt, but also for the values that students acquire during their training. It is well recognized that there is a hidden curriculum in medical education that impacts powerfully on students' ethical awareness. For example, medical students who learn how to be doctors in impersonal hospital bureaucracies sometimes take from those bureaucracies values which emphasize curing the disease at the price of alleviating the patient's suffering. Andre notes that students' developing 'ability to see the moral landscape' is constrained by a number of factors. She cites the stress and suffering and the 'sometimes desperate lack of time' during medical training as obstacles to clear moral vision (Andre 1992). Students who are occupied for most of the day in lectures, tutorials, and ward rounds and overwhelmed and exhausted by the volume of material to be learnt, are too tired, both physically and emotionally, to reflect on what it is that might make a good doctor.

Just as our characters are shaped by the social and cultural environment around us, so we are able to shape that environment ourselves. Our characters can and do contribute to social values and to the moral life of institutions. This is obvious when we meet individuals whose honesty and integrity have exercised a significant influence on the ethos of their work place. For example, many doctors will describe eloquently how, as medical students or junior doctors, their beliefs and values were shaped by their contact with consultants who, through example, exemplified for them what being a good doctor was all about. We might hope that, in a similar way, Dr Bowler's belief in the essential equality of human beings and his commitment to helping people might rub off on Imogen Jones.

Conclusion: what makes a good GP?

We began this chapter with the question: 'What makes a good general practitioner?' Throughout this book, we have tried to address this question in various ways. We have suggested that the good GP is trustworthy, discrete, beneficent, respectful, honest, fair, and compassionate. A critic might respond to this list by saying that these virtues ought to be upheld by *all* doctors. Are there virtues that are peculiar to general practice? Our answer to this question is that general practice does not have an exclusive claim to particular virtues. However, there are some virtues that seem particularly appropriate in a general practice context. In this concluding section, we return to the definition of general practice we offered in Chapter 1 and use it to sketch out some virtues for general practice.

General practice is distinguished by the central place it gives to the doctor–patient relationship. A number of things flow from this relationship—commitment to the patient as a whole human being, continuity of care over time, comprehensive care, and awareness of the patient's place in his or her family and wider community. These characteristics of relationships in general practice in turn suggest particular virtues.

Commitment to the patient as a person involves knowing and understanding the medical, personal, social, and psychological circumstances of one's patients. Jackie Silvers, in Chapter 1, was a beneficiary of her GP's commitment to her as a person.

Case 10.3

Ms Jackie Silvers is a 35-year-old mother of three young children. She lives with her husband who is an executive with a computer company and who spends a lot of time away from home. Their youngest child has severe asthma, and the middle child has extremely aggressive behaviour that has responded only poorly to a series of appointments with a psychologist. Ms Silvers presents on this occasion with recurrent headaches. Dr Whittaker knows that her husband is away in the USA on a three week trip, and that the youngest child was admitted last week as an emergency with his asthma. Ms Silvers has recently had a promotion in her work and is now managing a team of staff in the local council offices.

Dr Whittaker takes a history and examines Ms Silvers. His provisional diagnosis is that these are tension headaches, exacerbated by recent stresses in Ms Silvers' life.

Dr Whittaker's knowledge of Ms Silvers as a person helps him to reach a diagnosis and to spare Ms Silvers the inconvenience and anxiety of further investigations. His contact with Ms Silvers involves both action and promise (May 1994). Dr Whittaker's actions involve taking a thorough history and conducting a careful examination. His promises may be various, depending on what he feels is appropriate therapeutically and what Ms Silvers wishes—"There are a number of things we can do to help you", "I can assure you that this is nothing serious". Such promises are worthless if Dr Whittaker does not follow them through. Therefore, the virtue that Dr Whittaker needs to practise here is fidelity, the virtue of being true to one's promises, which is an important part of being trustworthy. And being true to one's promises acquires special poignancy in general practice, because relationships can often last a long time.

The length of relationship between doctor and patient is associated with a second characteristic of general practice—the provision of continuous care. Because GPs provide continuity of care over time they need the virtue of perseverance. Perseverance has at least two facets: it involves the capacity to pursue diligently the concerns that the patient brings, and it requires persistence to stick with a patient when things do not seem to go right. The specialist may return a patient to a GP with the words: "I can't find anything wrong here", but the GP does not have this luxury. His role as the point of continuing contact means that he can not wash his hands of his patients. May suggests that such behaviour is one of the 'inconspicuous marks of courage' (May 1994, p. 86), for perseverance requires that we continue in the face of adversity. In Dr Whittaker's case, adversity may show its face in the fact that he is unable to do more than offer band aid solutions to Ms Silvers' problems. Ms Silvers may be a difficult and demanding patient, who implies that Dr Whittaker ought to be able to do more for her. It may require considerable perseverence to continue to care for such a patient.

The third characteristic of relationships in general practice is the comprehensiveness of the care required. GPs must be able to see anything that walks in the door. There are many virtues associated with good comprehensive care—conscientiousness, perseverance, and prudence all spring to mind. One virtue that is often forgotten here is the virtue of humility. The lengthy training and specialized knowledge that accompanies being a doctor often brings with it a sense of superiority and patients may pander to this in many ways. Yet, virtuous practice acknowledges, as Dr Bowler does at the beginning of this chapter, that there is nothing inherently 'special' about the knowledge and skills of the doctor. The virtuous GP recognizes that people are 'all the same, underneath' and this underpins the attitude of respectfulness that the good GP brings to her work.

Finally, general practice locates patients in the context of their whole lives and acknowledges that patients are, first and foremost, people with hopes, fears, and ongoing lives. GPs, more than any other specialty in medicine, have the opportunity to practise the virtues of ordinary, everyday life—trustworthiness, thoughtfulness, patience, generosity, integrity. The list here is endless, but the point of the list is important. At the end of the day, the good GP is a good human being, practising the virtues in a particular setting with the special responsibilities and joys that this brings.

References

Andre, J. (1992). Learning to see: moral growth during medical training. *Journal of Medical Ethics* **18**, 148–52.

Blum, L. (1997). Compassion. In Kruschwitz, R.C. and Roberts, R.B. (ed.) *The virtues. Contemporary essays on moral character*, pp. 229–38. Wadsworth Publishing Company, Belmont, CA.

Brody, H. (1998). The family physician: what sort of person? *Family Medicine* **30** (8) 589–93.

Drane, J.F. (1994). Character and the moral life. A virtue approach to biomedical ethics. In DuBose, E.R., Hamel, R., and O'Connell, L.J. (ed.) *A matter of principles? Ferment in US bioethics*, pp. 284–309. Trinity Press International, valley Forge, PA.

May, W. (1994). The virtues in a professional setting. In Fulford, K.W.M., Gillett, G.R., and Soskice, J.M. (ed.) *Medicine and moral reasoning*, pp. 75–90. Cambridge University Press, Cambridge.

Nussbaum, M. (1996). Compassion: the basic social emotion. *Social Philosophy and Policy* **13**, 27–58.

Pellegrino, E.D. (1995). Toward a virtue-based normative ethics for the health professions. *Kennedy Institute of Ethics Journal* **5**, 253–60.

Veatch, R.M. (1985). Against virtue—a deontological critique of virtue theory in medical ethics. In Shelp, E.E. (ed.) *Virtue and medicine*, pp. 329–45. D Reidel Publishing Company, Boston, MA.

Further reading

Andre, J. (1992). Learning to see: moral growth during medical training. *Journal of Medical Ethics* **18**, 148–52.

Brody, H. (1998). The family physician: What sort of person? *Family Medicine* **30**, 589–93.

May, W. (1994). The virtues in a professional setting. In Fulford, K.W.M., GilleH, G.R., and Soskice, J.M. (ed.), pp. 75–90, *Medical and moral reasoning*. Cambridge University Press, Cambridge.

Pellegrino, E.D. and Thomasma, D.C. (1993). *The virtues in medical practice*. Oxford University Press, New York, NY.

Toon, P. (1999). *Towards a philosophy of general practice: the virtuous practitioner*. RCGP occasional papers 78. RCGP, London.

General reading and resources for medical ethics

Books

Beauchamp, T.L. and Childress, J.F. (2001). *Principles of biomedical ethics*, (5th edn). Oxford University Press, New York, NY.

Campbell, A., Gillett, G. and Jones, G. (2001). *Medical ethics* (3rd edn). Oxford University Press, Oxford.

Christie, R.J. and Hoffmaster, C.B. (1986). *Ethical issues in family medicine*. Oxford University Press, New York, NY.

Gillon, R. (1986). *Philosophical medical ethics*. John Wiley and sons, Chichester.

Mason, J. and McCall Smith, R. (2002). *Law and medical ethics* (6th edn). Butterworths, London.

Parker, M. and Dickenson, D. (ed.) (2001). *The Cambridge medical ethics workbook*. Cambridge University Press, Cambridge.

Singer, P.A. (ed.) (1999). *Bioethics at the beside: a clinician's guide*. Canadian Medical Association, Ottawa. Also published as *Canadian Medical Association Journal Bioethics for Clinicians Series*. Available from *http://www.cmaj.ca/cgi/collection/bioethics for clinicians series*

Sugarman, J. (ed.) (2000). *20 common problems—ethics in primary care*. McGraw-Hill, New York, NY.

Websites

Bioethics line. This dedicated bioethics database is accessed via the National Library of Medicine Gateway page. To search Bioethics line, click 'Limits' fom the menu on the opening page. Then select 'Bioethics' from the drop-down menu in the subsets box on the next page, and proceed with search. *http://gateway.nlm.nih.gov/gw/Cmd*

British Medical Association. The BMA provides a series of publications related to ethics. These can be accessed from the menu on the left hand side of the main home page. *http://www.bma.org.uk/*

Central Office for Research Ethics Committees. COREC is the central coordinating body for all research ethics committees in the UK. The website provides information on the role of ethics committees and how to prepare and submit applications. *http://www.corec.org*

General Medical Council. The GMC provides a range of guidance as well as specific publications on ethical issues. These can be accessed by following the links to ethical guidance from the menu bar on the main home page. *http://www.gmc-uk.org/index.htm*

Internet Encyclopaedia of Philosophy. The IEP is an on-line encyclopaedia providing entries on a wide range of topics including ethics. *http://www.utm.edu/research/iep/*

Journal of Medical Ethics. The JME is a bi-monthly journal that publishes articles on a wide range of medical ethics topics, including research, health care practice, and conceptual analysis. *http://jme.bmjjournals.com/*

National Bioethics Advisory Commission Publications. These reports and commissioned papers from the USA focus mainly on research with humans, and include topics such as cloning and stem cell research. They are available from Georgetown University website: *http://bioethics.georgetown.edu/nbac/pubs.html*

World Medical Association. The WMA has a new Ethics Unit with information about and access to a variety of publications and resources on medical ethics and related topics. The website is new and some areas are under development. The Ethics Unit can be accessed from the menu on the left hand side of the WMA main page. *http://www.wma.net/e/*

Index